Autism and Anxiety

By

Charlotte Chaney &
Danielle Punter

Autability offers a selection of training materials which are accredited by
The CPD Standards Authority.

CPD Provider: 50373

For more information on books and training materials which are currently accredited, please visit
www.autability.co.uk/programlist

Other books Charlotte Chaney & Danielle Punter

Parenting Rewired:
How to raise a happy autistic child in a very neurotypical world

ISBN 978 1 83997 072 6
eISBN 978 1 83997 073 3

For those professionals who helped
Kiddo through the toughest of times.

With thanks to our Autability medical team.

CONTENTS

INTRODUCTION

Welcome to our second book!

We are Charlotte and Danielle, co-directors of Autability and diagnosed neurodivergent parents to our amazing neurodivergent children.

We began writing together in 2021. Our first book, 'Parenting Rewired: How to raise a happy autistic child in a very neurotypical world', was published in 2022. Since then we have developed a training company, aimed at parents and professionals, who want to understand the autistic and ADHD mind and change their patterns of behaviour to allow the child or young person to flourish as who they really are.

We are privileged to have two experienced psychiatrists and a neurodivergent consultant on our team. They check our content for medical accuracy. To us, this is important as it gives our work legitimacy, especially when used by professionals. To find out more about our own experiences, both at work and at home, head over to www.autability.co.uk and see what we do.

This book wasn't formally planned, it happened by accident. The challenging journey to get appropriate help for autistic people who suffer from anxiety is no secret, especially when it relates to children and young people. Danielle was keen to write about her own experiences as a teenager and also those of her son (who is called "Kiddo" throughout this book), who at age 8, was diagnosed with Generalised Anxiety Disorder (GAD). Kiddo also has diagnoses of autism and ADHD and struggles with verbal communication, relying on echolalia a great deal. Being diagnosed with GAD, depression and ADHD herself, Danielle has experienced the UK medical system as both a patient under the age of 18 and as a parent/carer. Helpful resources for parents desperately trying to support their children through anxious times aren't always readily available. This places huge pressure on family relationships, as parents and professionals search for ways to help children and young people overcome their anxieties.

Charlotte has extensive experience with mental health support services through her son (who is called "Pie" throughout this book) and has seen the best and worst in terms of provision, support and medical services. Pie has several psychological diagnoses including severe clinical depression and psychosis presenting with ocular and auditory hallucinations. In addition, Pie has an acquired brain injury which impacts on his mental health. Charlotte was diagnosed with depression and anxiety as a teenager, presentations which still exist to this day. Charlotte is diagnosed autistic and ADHD and writes about her experiences as a child and how the neurotypical world can automatically induce anxiety for a neurodivergent person.

A question we are constantly asked is, "can an autistic person suffer from anxiety? Or is it just their autism?" In short, the answer is yes they can. However, parents and professionals must understand where the difference lies in terms of the need for medication and therapeutic interventions. In the first chapter, we explain this in detail and hopefully will give you an idea of what type of help your child/young person/student needs.

Whether someone requires professional help or not, there is still a huge amount that can be done by parents and front-line professionals to help autistic children and young people. The difficulty is finding a resource that gives enough understanding and detail. Upon realising this we decided a guide was needed, especially for those who, for whatever reason, cannot get access to child and adolescent mental health services where they are.

As always, our writing may challenge you or perhaps ask you to consider a different viewpoint. We don't do this because we believe we are right and everyone else is wrong. We do it to give you, the reader, a genuine insight into the working of the autistic brain and how such small changes can make important differences in the quality of life for an autistic person. You may not understand why the change that occurs is so significant, but you don't have to. Neurotypical and neurodivergent brains work differently. It's only by accepting this and learning how a brain wired differently to our own brain works, that we can make huge strides for our children and create a world that celebrates them for who they really are.

This book will not tell you you're wrong, or you've failed. We are here to give you hope and encouragement when you just can't see a way forward.

We hope it helps.

CHAPTER ONE

"Let's start at the very beginning...."

Before you start this book, it's important you know exactly what we mean by 'anxiety', 'autism' and various other terms. In this opening chapter, we will look at various diagnoses and explain why they do, or don't, fit with the type of anxiety we will be concentrating on. So please don't skip this chapter, it's information we all need to know!

What is autism?

A common myth about autism is that it is a mental health condition. It isn't. It is a neurodevelopmental condition, which is completely different.

A neurodevelopmental condition shows up in the development period and is often characterised by impairment in social, academic or occupational functioning.

A mental health condition (or disorder) is, "characterised by a clinically significant disturbance in an individual's cognition, emotional regulation, or behaviour."[1]

Autism is, "characterised by persistent deficits in social communication and social interaction across multiple contexts, including deficits in social reciprocity, non-verbal communicative behaviours used for social interaction, and skills in developing, maintaining and understanding relationships."[2] The diagnostic criteria also specify the presence of repetitive behaviours and some sensory challenges.

We see that autism alone could technically fit into both categories. However, what causes autism to present as a disturbance in cognition, emotional regulation and behaviour (mental health condition) is having to conform to a neurotypical way of life. Without these pressures, and with encouragement to be the person you are, autism should only present as a different way of social functioning. Sadly, this world often forces autistic people to conform to a way of behaviour which prevents them from regulating emotionally and physically and it is here we see the onset of mental health conditions. One of the most common mental health conditions experienced by autistic people is anxiety.

---

[1] World Health Organisation, www.who.int/news-room/fact-sheets/detail/mental-disorders

[2] Diagnostic and Statistical Manual of Mental Disorders, fifth edition, DSM V 2013

What is anxiety?

One of the big problems with anxiety is that the words 'anxious' and 'anxiety' are words used in everyday language to describe perfectly normal and healthy human emotions. Feeling 'anxious' or 'nervous' can be beneficial. For example, it can encourage a person to push themselves that little bit further and discover new experiences. When a child starts a new school, or an adult starts a new job, butterflies in the tummy are completely normal. Such everyday normalising of the word 'anxiety' means it can be difficult for people without a formal diagnosis to perceive anxiety as a diagnosed mental health disorder. The anxiety we are talking about in this guide is the clinical condition known as 'Generalised Anxiety Disorder' (GAD).

The DSM V defines GAD as, "excessive anxiety and worry (apprehensive expectation), occurring more days than not for at least 6 months, about a number of events or activities (such as work or school performance). The individual finds it difficult to control the worry."[3]

The DSM also lists specific symptoms associated with worry or anxiety. Of the following, one must be present for a child to receive a diagnosis and three for an adult:

- Restlessness or feeling keyed up or on edge
- Being easily fatigued

[3] Diagnostic and Statistical Manual of Mental Disorders, fifth edition, DSM V 2013

- Difficulty concentrating or mind going blank
- Irritability
- Muscle tension
- Sleep disturbance (difficulty falling or staying asleep, or restless, unsatisfying sleep)

Finally, the anxiety, worry, or physical symptoms cause clinically significant distress or impairment in social, occupational, or other important areas of functioning. Some people will experience multiple symptoms, whilst others may only experience one or two. The severity of anxiety isn't gauged by the number of symptoms but rather by the impact such symptoms have on a person's daily living. So, is the issue 'normal' levels of nerves and worries, which are a part of everyday life? Or a level of anxiety that needs to be considered for a clinical diagnosis? We've listed the differences in a table for you to compare.

Non-pathological anxiety	Generalised Anxiety Disorder
Worries of everyday life not excessive Worries perceived as more manageable Worries can be put off when more pressing worries arise	Worries are excessive Worries interfere with psychosocial functioning
Worries are less pervasive and distressing Worries have a shorter duration Worries don't occur very often	Worries are more pervasive, pronounced and distressing Worries are longer in duration Worries occur frequently

Everyday worries are not accompanied by physical symptoms	Worries cause impairment in social, occupational and other important areas of functioning
Anxiety NOT accompanied by: Restlessness Feeling keyed up Fatigue Difficulty concentrating Mind going blank Irritability Muscle tension Disturbed sleep	Anxiety accompanied by ONE of the following for children, or THREE of the following for adults : Restlessness Feeling keyed up Fatigue Difficulty concentrating Mind going blank Irritability Muscle tension Disturbed sleep

There are some conditions that people commonly associate with anxiety but are separate. We've listed some below, and let you know whether or not they are covered in this book.

Condition/ Illness	**What is it?**	**How does it differ to GAD?**
Post Traumatic Stress Disorder (PTSD)	The anxiety is in response to an identifiable stressor It does not persist for more than6 months after the termination of the stressor or it's consequences	GAD is excessive worry which is always present PTSD is a reaction which ONLY occurs when the person is triggered by a specific stressor(s) This book DOES NOT discuss PTSD

Obsessive Compulsive Disorder (OCD)	Inappropriate obsessions and ideas that take the form of intrusive and unwanted thoughts, urges or images	OCD is NOT excessive worry about future events which is abnormal This book DOES NOT discuss OCD
Social Anxiety Disorder	Anticipatory anxiety that is focused on upcoming social situations in which they must perform or be evaluated	Those with GAD worry about social situations whether they are being evaluated or not. This book DOES discuss some features of Social Anxiety Disorder
Depression and bipolar disorders	Generalised anxiety is a common feature of both GAD is usually not diagnosed if depression or bipolar is present	This book DOES discuss features of depression and bipolar where anxiety is also present

Is anxiety common in autistic people?

Getting a precise statistic of how many autistic people suffer from clinical anxiety is difficult as there are so many studies with their statistics. A study carried out in 2021 by Julia Forte at Stranmillis University in Belfast, investigated the prevalence of anxiety in autistic children compared to typically developing children. The respondents in this study were parents of autistic and typically developing children, 75% of parents with an autistic child responded that their child regularly experienced anxiety compared to just 11% of typically developing children. The actual prevalence of autistic people who experience anxiety is most likely much higher. There will be those autistic children who are unable to communicate they are feeling anxious and those who do not have interoceptive abilities, which identify these physical feelings. Interoception is the ability to understand the signals your body is sending. For example, if you are hungry your tummy may rumble, which means hunger and you respond by eating. Many autistic children and adults can struggle to interpret such signals. In the case of anxiety in children, this means they are often unable to express what they are experiencing. They may also mask their anxiety, meaning their parents/carers are unaware.

Does autism cause anxiety?

Whilst anxiety is not currently listed as a diagnostic criterion for autism, the figures above confirm anxiety is common among autistic children (and adults). There is no known underlying biological reason why an autistic person is more likely to experience clinical anxiety. However, when you look at the challenges which an autistic person deals with daily, it is evident why there is such a high level of anxious autistics.

Dealing with unpredictable sensory environments is a major contributor to creating anxiety in autistic people. Needing to interact and be in social situations is also anxiety-inducing, as autistic people often struggle to be understood or accepted by neurotypical peers. It is as though you are trying to fit a square peg (the autistic person) into a round hole (the neurotypical world). It doesn't fit, yet instead of changing the shape of the hole, most concentrate on changing the shape of the person and that often produces high levels of anxiety.

We examine different areas where anxiety can negatively impact an autistic person. There will always be elements of sensory, social and communication in each of these areas.

Environmental anxiety triggers can also cause anxiety in neurotypical people and shouldn't be seen as 'autistic only' causes. The same can be said for chemical imbalances in the brain, which can mean a person is more likely to struggle with clinical anxiety. Being autistic doesn't make a person more or less likely to present these imbalances. There are several chemicals and neurotransmitters which can cause anxiety with the most well-known being serotonin. Whilst low serotonin is known to cause anxiety, being anxious also lowers your serotonin levels.

Alexythmia and anxiety

As we have already discussed, anxiety is an emotion, characterised by feelings of tension, worry and physical changes. The inability to understand and regulate emotion is a common experience for many autistic people. Some have a condition called alexithymia.

Alexithymia is defined in the DSM V as, "deficits in cognitive processing of emotions".[4] In simple terms it means, "no

---

[4] Diagnostic and Statistical manual of mental disorders fifth edition DSM V 2013

words for emotion".[5] It can also mean a person struggles to sense physical symptoms, such as a change in heart rate.

Alexithymia, along with interoceptive difficulties, can mean an autistic person is unable to identify the physical or emotional symptoms of anxiety. A further consideration is when an autistic person is unable to regulate their emotions. If you're feeling strange and you don't know why, it can be terrifying. You know you need to alter the state you are in, but how can you fix it when you don't know what the problem is? The capacity to identify emotions and physical symptoms is key to remaining calm and regulated, whilst meeting your own needs. Without that capability or the help of anyone else who has learnt to read the signs of such dysregulation, anxiety builds as you may be unaware of when these feelings will strike and how to handle them.

Therapeutic interventions

Some autistic children and young people are offered talking therapies to reduce their anxiety. There are various options, including CBT (Cognitive Behavioural Therapy), exposure therapy (therapies to break the patterns of fear and avoidance), mindfulness techniques, and sensory integration training (helping children to use all their senses together). These can be effective for some autistic children and young people and they must be delivered by an accredited practitioner with an understanding and knowledge of autism.

5 www.autistica.org.uk/what-is-autism/anxiety-and-autism-hub/alexithymia

For adults in England, there is statutory guidance that states that an autistic adult with mental health difficulties must have access to support which is adapted to their needs. Currently no such guidance exists for those under eighteen.

If your child has alexithymia, you must make this known to any therapist or professional working on supporting your child's anxiety. Alexithymia will have a profound impact on the effectiveness of certain therapies and therapy may need to be approached differently. Children and young people who have alexithymia may need to begin with support in understanding and identifying their emotions and communicating their feelings before engaging in more specific anxiety-reducing therapy.

It is important to note that, whilst anxiety can reduce serotonin levels, reducing anxiety will in turn increase serotonin levels. The effect of therapies when treating anxiety in autistic children and young people is dependent upon many factors. These include communication abilities and profiles, tolerance to sensory stimuli, the ability to process thoughts and feelings when in the company of other people and the ability to visualise themselves in different situations. All of these factors mean that for some autistic people, talking therapies may never be an option, whilst others may need medication to be able to engage with it. For some it works fantastically and talking therapy should always be a primary consideration in the treatment of anxiety in autistic people, with an appropriately qualified therapist.

Medical interventions

Thankfully the taboo surrounding anti-depressant medication has diminished over the past three decades. People no longer secretly ingest their "happy pills", dreading the discussion that may happen if someone was to find out what they were taking. With this acceptance can also come a complacency that anxiety can be "cured" with medication.

Add autism into the mix and the picture surrounding whether a person needs medication becomes even more controversial and confusing. What is important is that, whilst being furnished with an understanding of how these drugs work, there are several factors to be considered on an individual basis by a child and adolescent psychiatrist, before prescribing any medication to treat anxiety.

Most anti-depressants and anti-anxiety medications work by increasing the brain's serotonin level. As previously mentioned, low levels of serotonin cause anxiety, meaning some people are genetically predisposed to anxiety. Here, serotonin-increasing medication is likely to have a positive impact on clinical anxiety.

Many psychiatrists are cautious in prescribing medication to mitigate anxiety in an autistic child or young person. They often work on the assumption that the anxiety is caused by environmental triggers which are heightened by autism. If you think your child needs drug therapy to improve their anxiety, it is worth reminding the psychiatrist that anxiety can cause low levels of serotonin, even in a person who is not predisposed to clinical anxiety. This means a person in this category may also respond well to serotonin-increasing medication.

Medication can be used as a short-term measure to enable a person to control their anxiety to the point where they can access other interventions to support them. However, medication is rarely a game changer by itself. Lots of support is required from parents, family, friends and professionals once the child is at a point where they can access environments that once they were not. The child will need a chance to build up their confidence, learn new ways of thinking (where appropriate) and form trusting relationships with those around them. Medication is only the beginning.

Getting support

There are many self-help ideas that you can implement to support your autistic child with anxiety. We will discuss some of these in more detail later in this book. Self-help ideas can include adding structure to your autistic child's day, helping their sensory regulation and supporting their communication and social skills. For some, this may be life-changing and mean their anxiety no longer impacts their life in the same negative way. For others, there may be no change and specialist medical support and help are required.

Accessing child and young person's mental health services (CAMHS) is becoming increasingly difficult. Accessing child and young person's mental health services for an autistic child is for most a time-consuming and emotionally draining battle. This is due to local teams often using their own specific criteria for autistic children and young people. The wording may alter from service to service but in a nutshell, autistic children can only access these services if there is clear evidence that their anxiety/ depression is not caused by their autism.

A frequent and justified question from parents is, "How do we do that?"

Sadly, there is often no definitive answer. Charlotte's autistic son, Pie, was first referred to CAMHS when he was six. He was presenting not with anxiety but with a very low mood and his paediatrician was concerned. Despite the paediatrician's best efforts, initial attempts to be seen by CAMHS were fruitless. Pie's presentation was further complicated when he began having visual and auditory hallucinations. This was all happening whilst he was receiving no specialist care. He was prescribed a sedative by an emergency GP and he was referred to the crisis team. Despite multiple phone calls a day, it took 23 working days for him to be assessed. Once assessed it took less than 23 minutes for him to be put on anti-depressants and anti-psychotic medication. Since then, Charlotte can't fault the service they have received from their local CAMHS or the two London CAMHS teams. What does upset Charlotte deeply is that in the ten years since Pie was first seen and accepted by CAMHS, there has been no improvement in the care and support offered to autistic children in the UK.

This has been proven by Danielle's recent 4-year battle to get her son, Kiddo, even assessed by a psychiatrist on the NHS.

She provided evidence that everything that could be done to reduce anxiety as a result of being autistic and living in a neurotypical world, was currently being done. She had a family history of anxiety and Danielle herself was even diagnosed with Generalised Anxiety Disorder. It took fight after fight and formal procedures to even get a psychiatrist to visit and assess Kiddo. When someone did finally agree, it was clear to them he was suffering from an additional anxiety disorder, which was separate from his autism. Along with Kiddo's school, Danielle was able to show how much had already been put in place and that with Kiddo's communication difficulties, talking therapies were not an option. He was diagnosed with Generalised Anxiety Disorder and given completely life-changing medication. There is no doubt that Kiddo's health, education and social skills, hugely suffered during this time, as did the mental health of Danielle and Kiddo's Dad. This is a key reason why we encourage all parents to put in place any support they can themselves before pursuing a long battle which has no guarantees. The more you can evidence of what has been put in place to support your autistic child at home and school, the more likely a psychiatrist is to consider there may be an additional problem. For more information on how to support your autistic child in everyday life, see our book, 'Parenting Rewired[6].

So, whilst being autistic can increase your chances of experiencing anxiety, an autistic person can also have a separate anxiety disorder and/or mental health condition.

---

6 www.autability.co.uk/parentingrewired

CHAPTER TWO

Sensory Processing and Anxiety

It is estimated approximately 90% of autistic people also have sensory processing difficulties.[7] Not everyone with sensory processing disorder will experience anxiety, but having sensory processing difficulties will increase your autistic child's likelihood of experiencing clinical anxiety.

Sensory processing disorder (SPD) can cause a person to feel overwhelmed and in turn this heightened state makes it harder to regulate and reduce anxiety triggers. Our senses are working 24/7 and this means some individuals with SPD will be dealing with triggering sensory input constantly. It can impact multiple areas of their lives from going to busy places, attending school, trying new food, personal hygiene, getting dressed and sleeping.

I have heard neurotypical people complain if a light is too bright or positioned wrongly, requesting (often in an

---

7 https://www.ncbi.nlm.nih.gov/pmc/articles/PMC3086654/

abrupt manner) that the light be switched off. Perhaps they complain about the sound of chalk squeaking on a board, or not like the feel of a particular garment. For most people, these unpopular sensations are no more than a minor inconvenience. The light can be turned off, the chalk squeak will end after a couple of seconds and there are plenty of garments in your wardrobe that you like the feel of.

Imagine if that light couldn't be switched off and at the same time you were being subjected to a person deliberately squeaking chalk on the blackboard, all whilst wearing a head-to-toe garment made of a fabric that you found uncomfortable? Add in some strong offensive smells and an enclosed space for good measure and you have an idea of how it feels to have a sensory processing disorder.

Few people relish the sensations being described. Well, things are about to get worse. In addition, your ability to verbally communicate your feelings is taken away, and you can't get the triggers reversed. These feelings are going to re-occur in various intensities and combinations throughout your day. With no notice, your sensory system will overload with a booming fanfare. It'll never be the same type of overload twice, meaning there is little you can do to overcome your brain's response.

How does sensory overload make us anxious?

Although the experience of sensory overload is unpleasant, to say the least, why would something many autistic people experience every day create such feelings of anxiety?

Ask yourself, would you watch a horror film when you are already on edge? No, because it would frighten you. Fear makes us anxious. It puts us on edge and releases hormones designed to protect us in situations our bodies and brains perceive as dangerous. Imagine facing every single day with the alarm going off in your head that danger is everywhere from the minute you wake up, you're hardly going to be feeling calm and collected. So why are sensory overloads feared by autistic people? We've listed a few reasons:

- No two sensory experiences are the same. You can't plan how to regulate each overload. You're at the mercy of your environment and are constantly scanning for things which might trigger overload. Anything could be a threat.
- The fear of having a meltdown in public, especially when you're school-age, is terrifying. You can't control a meltdown. Once it starts you are powerless to stop it. It makes you vulnerable in social situations where you are likely already masking, trying to fit in and go unnoticed.
- Anxiety about the pain you feel in your head from sensory overload can be all-encompassing. It may be different each time, but it's not positive. It's not something you want to experience so you avoid it and become worried about experiencing it. If you get hit by a car and injured, you're likely to be extra cautious and anxious around moving cars, especially in the days following the incident. The anxiety around the pain of overload is no different.

We hope this description is enough to ensure that even the most sensory-regulated reader amongst you will have no difficulty in understanding how sensory processing can trigger anxiety. Also, we hope it shows how that anxiety can be triggered by a seemingly insignificant sensory input. Anxiety is a cumulative response that builds over time, not from a single sensory input, but several inputs.

Sensory solutions

There is no general off switch to sensory input. Sensory stimulation is everywhere. Sitting writing this, Charlotte is trying not to be triggered by her Labrador's roaring snore or the landing light which is shining under her bedroom door. We know that we can't prevent these. For Charlotte, this knowledge comes from four decades of exposure to unwanted sensory input.

Charlotte knows the weighted blanket she is wrapped in helps her regulate, as does stroking her snoring (or otherwise) Labrador or cats. Her brain is still being made to process the unwanted invasion of sensory input but is regulating and reducing the negative sensations via these two positive sensory inputs.

How each person processes sensory input and output is constantly fluid. No two sensory experiences are the same. This doesn't mean there won't be "go-to" solutions for your child, it just takes a long time to learn what these are.

How to discover what works

Understanding your child's sensory profile is essential to helping them remain regulated, calm and content. Here are some areas to take note of when observing your child, followed by a diary template which you can use over several weeks to get a clearer idea of how your child is feeling and what they are struggling to process.

What to look for:

- Are there any days of the week which have the same behavioural pattern? For example, if your child is dysregulated every Wednesday in the same way, what might be causing it? Look for activities and routines on Tuesday, Wednesday and Thursday. The struggles may not be related to the actual day they present themselves. They could be processing an activity that regularly happens the previous day or the next day.
- Note any activities where your child is calm. This includes before, during and after the activity. For example, are they calm when running? This may mean they need vestibular input. Are they calm when doing tactile activities with a particular material? This could help with touch and proprioception. Noting the material is essential, as the difference between using Play-Doh and sand could be significant.

- Are there any activities your child loves to do, but struggle to calm down from afterwards? Many children can become overstimulated by an activity they love, so it is important to keep a record of how long they can stay regulated before they start experiencing overload. You can have too much of a good thing.
- Are there specific foods that calm your child down? Are they chewy? Hot? Cold? Rough? Smooth? This will help you understand more about the sensations they crave to regulate.
- Is there a theme with the activities that can make your child feel distressed? For example, if you go to different venues and your child copes with some and not others, what are the common factors? Is it noisy? Bright? Crowded? It may not be the venue itself, but the sensory differences caused by the number of people etc.
- Does your child notice when they are hungry, thirsty or need the toilet? Or is it a sudden desperate need? It could be they have poor interoception and can't feel their body's cues when it needs something. The sudden feeling of hunger, for example, can make a child feel distressed.
- Are there areas of the house they stay away from? Or areas they often seek out? For example, are the smells from the kitchen too much?

Figure 1. shows an example of the sheet partially filled in. You can find this template for free on our website here: https://www.autability.co.uk/product-page/sensory-diary-sheet

Use the diary sheet to make a note of moods, behaviours and activities over a long period. This information will be key to supporting your child. For more information, www.autability.co.uk or see our book, "Parenting Rewired – how to raise a happy autistic child in a very neurotypical world".

Figure 1

Day	Time	Event/Activity	Calm	Distressed	Over excited	Other /notes
Mon	4pm	Changing out of school uniform		✓		Bad day at school
Sat	11am	Trampolining			✓	Couldn't calm down after being on the trampoline

CHAPTER THREE

Anxiety and School

Anxiety around school is one of the most well known issues when raising an autistic child. Terms such as 'school refusal' are thrown around and you often hear of parents fighting for schools and provisions to make reasonable adaptations, so a neurodivergent pupil can have the best experience possible for them. What is often missed is a deeper explanation as to why these children and young people find school so anxiety-inducing. We've selected a few reasons for this chapter, as it is only by understanding why someone finds an experience anxiety-provoking that we can make effective changes for them.

The pressure to communicate

You learnt French at school. You haven't studied French for 12 years but end up on holiday in France with your family. You're in a restaurant where there is no English spoken and no English language menus. Your entire family is relying on you to translate and order for them. How would you feel? Stressed – anxious – pressured to name a few things!

This is an easy way to describe how hard it can be for an autistic child in the classroom. There is constant expectation and pressure to be able to communicate. There is an expected protocol of communication in the classroom.

From a teaching perspective, communication is a crucial ingredient to a good teaching style. A teacher will be aware of the communication skills of their class. The communication style will be more formal between adult and pupil than it would be pupil to pupil. Often this makes it much easier for the child to predict what is required but also hopefully the communication will be scaffolded appropriately.

Talking to peers is a minefield. Vocabulary changes and there is a development of language skills and expectations. As the other pupils are also on their trajectory of language development it can mean that they will not have the ability or understanding to acknowledge that other children might be struggling, especially during primary school. By the time secondary school is reached, there is an even higher expectation and less parent expectation of how pupils will communicate both socially and in the classroom. If this is not met it can quickly become a cause of amusement, teasing and in some cases extend to bullying.

Danielle can remember starting secondary school and it was like entering a world where she needed to use a new language. During the first few days, a friend of hers asked her if she thought a boy in their class was "fit". She replied, "I don't know really, he was good at cross country in primary school". This caused several pupils to disintegrate into giggles with Danielle just looking at them bemused. Eventually one of them said, "you got confused! You thought I meant "fit" as in good at sport and I meant "fit" as in good looking!" At that moment Danielle realised how much she was going to have to re-learn. Danielle was easily able to stand up for herself and didn't experience bullying during school. For so many children though, this is not the case and the misunderstanding of language can be a basis on which teasing can begin.

The pressure of learning and managing several communication styles is one of the little-acknowledged causes of anxiety among children. It's not uncommon for this anxiety to manifest in selective mutism, social withdrawal and a decline in academic performance. If you are unsure of how your child copes with communication demands at school, it is worth talking to their teachers. If they are in primary school, you may also be able to observe their peer-on-peer interaction at school drop-off and collection.

Whilst anxiety which is induced by communication can of course impact any autistic child, it is important to note that the expectations can be much higher when a child is in a mainstream school.

Often simple support strategies can help enormously, including comms cards, texting and awareness among school staff that your child is struggling. They can then, for example, use individual whiteboards and ask children to write their answers rather than ask pupils to answer verbally.

So much time is spent focusing on verbal skills in autistic children when the problem is communication and the anxiety and stress this causes. Whilst communication is one area, don't underestimate the anxiety that this can create.

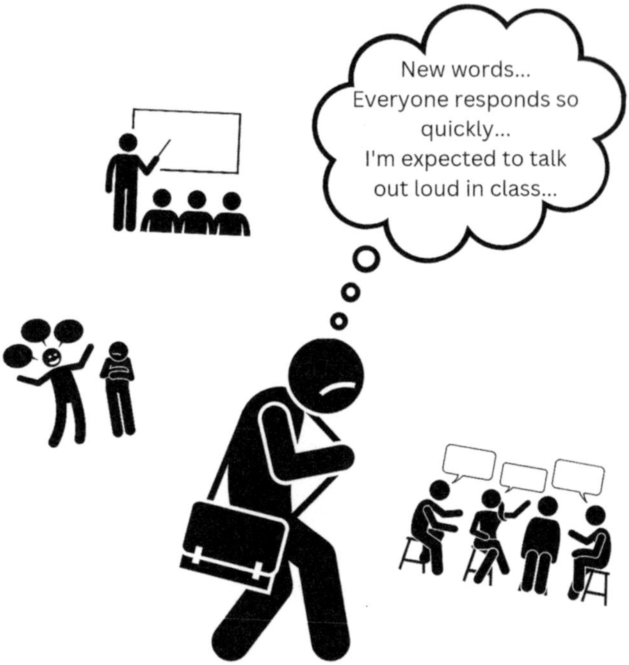
New words...
Everyone responds so quickly...
I'm expected to talk out loud in class...

Exams and academic achievement

One cause of anxiety in school children, especially those with additional needs, is around the academic areas that they struggle with. This is a massive and genuine issue, and we will cover it later in this chapter. But what about the child that overcomes hurdles and obstacles to attain high academic results, but sees themselves as a failure? This probably sounds crazy, but it happens. Charlotte has seen it happen to pupils she has taught, but her knowledge is even more personal because it happened to her.

At junior school, Charlotte struggled academically and socially but was fortunate in having a school that could see what her main obstacles were to learning. Whilst all her results were very low, it wasn't down to intellect, it was dyslexia and dyspraxia. Charlotte was fortunate to have the correct interventions at an early age. Gradually she started to be able to decipher words and whilst it took more energy and time, she was making progress. Her writing was poor but becoming legible and little by little she started to "catch up". In her head, Charlotte saw her learning as a ladder. The starting point was low. She was not even on the bottom step but little by little she started to make it upwards. Sometimes she would fall, but that seemed to make her more determined to climb. It was hard when she re-joined her chronological year group as the ladder climbing started at the bottom again. Unusually for Charlotte's brain, it seemed to go with it and with each laborious step, she learned a new technique to keep her scores where they should be. By the time she made the leap to Senior School Charlotte was average. In those days school reports would record the class average and the pupil average. Charlotte's score was always a little bit below or above the marker.

Charlotte loved senior school, there was more structure and depth to the learning which for the first time allowed her brain to explore what she now knows to be its' natural curiosity for information. She continued to progress and by the end of year 8, she came second in her year overall. A result which appeared to shock everyone, but nobody more than Charlotte. That year at prize giving she received two awards, one for second place and the whole school award for "consistent effort". This was the first time Charlotte had received any acknowledgement for academic work but this second award was, in fact, the start of anxiety being linked not to her schoolwork but to the outcome.

Charlotte felt that being awarded for her effort meant she had to try harder. She became obsessed with working. Charlotte would internalise her goals and strive for perfection. Nobody knew this was the case but to Charlotte, anything less than a top mark was a failure. She would worry and not sleep because sleep meant that she would miss out on some valuable learning opportunities.

Charlotte successfully managed to mask her anxiety and it went unnoticed. The remainder of her senior school years flew by and suddenly GCSEs were almost upon her. At age 7 a paediatrician suggested that Charlotte would be better suited to other assessments rather than GCSEs as they would be beyond her. Here she was at 15 with predicted grades of As and Bs yet anxious and worried about failure. The exams came and went, and Charlotte dealt with them in a methodical and unemotive manner. They were a process that she had to endure and whilst her peers seemed to be panicked, she just got on with it. Charlotte was more worried about results day. When it arrived she ripped open the envelope and all she saw was a failure. Charlotte knows if they were anyone else's results, she would have been overjoyed as she got nine As and one B. The B sent her spiralling. What could she have done to have got a B in geography? Should she have spent more time revising? What went wrong in her exam? She felt like a complete failure. Charlotte didn't even like geography, she had no intention of taking her learning of the subject any further. It was always an extra subject because she didn't want to have study lessons. Nothing was going to break this cycle. Charlotte refused any form of celebration or acknowledgement of what others perceived as a "success".

Charlotte wanted to hide from the world. She didn't know how this could have happened. Nobody could reason with her. If anybody else had got those results she would have been impressed, beyond impressed probably. But, in her head, she hadn't managed to fully overcome what she thought she had to.

Charlotte still has these thoughts today and Danielle has similar ones. Danielle's view of success and failure in school was very black-and-white. There was no in-between.

Danielle missed an A in one of her A levels by 1 mark, leaving her with two A's (the highest mark you could get) and one B. She got her place at University but the pain of that B was like a sharp stab to the chest because, in Danielle's mind, that was a failure. Exam results were all or nothing and it was a thought process Danielle couldn't and sometimes still can't help. For Danielle, the stress she carried surrounding exam results led her to be diagnosed with depression and anxiety whilst studying her A Levels. She became unable to take exams in the same hall as anyone else and hasn't sat a single exam in a large exam hall since she was 17.

For both Charlotte and Danielle, it is the way their brain functions and they can't change that.

What they have both learnt is how to have those feelings for less time and to process them. CBT was immensely helpful for Danielle with this, but for autistic people, CBT is a very individual experience.

When Charlotte began teaching, she was surprised to see how many children would respond similarly. What shocked her more was that it wasn't acknowledged as being a problem or a trigger of anxiety. In the early 2000s, there was more awareness made in education of the challenges of being "gifted and talented". But, there was a criterion to be put in this category and one which she wouldn't have fulfilled for academia. Overcoming hurdles and obstacles is part of daily life for neurodivergent people but sometimes we are unable to rationalise when we feel we are not doing as well as we perceive we should. So often parents say they don't understand why their child is anxious, especially if "they are doing well in school" but it is an area which is worth looking at, especially if your autistic child has made unexpected or more progress than anticipated.

The anxiety of no school

Home education and Education Other Than At School (EOTAS) is becoming a popular phenomenon amongst parents of children with SEND. Sometimes it is a voluntary decision and in other cases, it is the decision of the local authority, as they are unable to find a suitable placement. Before those of you who fall into the category throw away this book thinking we are about to criticise this – STOP – Charlotte deregistered her son from school when he was in year 2 and had a funded EOTAS for the past 7 years. For him this was the right decision, not because of his anxiety but other medical needs.

The common perception is that school is an anxiety trigger, so remove the trigger and the anxiety disappears. This theory could be applied to any anxiety trigger. Whilst it is logical, and in several cases true, for some the effect of removing school is detrimental. Here is an example of this:

F has a diagnosis of autism and Generalised Anxiety Disorder. F struggled at primary school and was given a place in a specialist ASD school for secondary. As F started secondary the pandemic hit and F had to shield. F had almost 18 months at home. F struggled with online learning but engaged with it. Once F was able to return to school in person it was not easy. F was determined to make it work. They made steady steps, which for F were giant leaps, but perceived by the school and local authority as minimal. F's steady progress was thrown off course by a school closure which hadn't been planned. The response of the school and the local authority was to terminate the placement and offer an EOTAS package. This was done without consultation with the parents and more importantly, F's views were not considered. In F's mind, school is what children and young people do. F wants to fit in. By removing the school placement, he perceives this as another sign that he is "different" to his perception of what is normal.

Whilst there is a reduction in F's anxiety relating to going out, as he doesn't have to process getting up and out to go to school, overall, there has been a massive detriment to F because he is unable to resolve the anger and feeling of grief at being refused a school place which has made his anxiety much worse.

When Kiddo was suffering from anxiety and was eventually diagnosed with Generalised Anxiety Disorder, he struggled to cope with the transition to and from school. Knowing how much Kiddo needed school, Danielle did everything she could to keep him going whilst she fought for medication (which isn't always necessary, but there were no changes left that the school could make to accommodate him and the school itself wasn't the cause).

He had a period where he struggled to attend school and not only did it make his world significantly smaller and isolate him further, it also made him feel extremely low. He is now back regularly and laughing and smiling! Removing school wasn't the answer, not for a long-term recovery where anxiety wouldn't affect him for the rest of his life. It was hard fighting for what Danielle knew he would need long term, so he could recover and manage his anxiety. It's very easy for services to look at the here and now, and in desperation parents remove the trigger altogether for some peace and recovery time. This may be necessary temporarily while the child recuperates, but it is so important to ask yourself if how you are planning to solve this problem in the immediate future is going to help your child long term. Sometimes the best remedy for anxiety is supporting your child to develop the resilience to work through their anxiety at their pace.

CHAPTER FOUR

Anxiety, Autism and Cognitive Functioning

Autism doesn't impact a person's intellect meaning that there will be autistic individuals with an entire spectrum of IQ range. Linking a person's intellect to anxiety may appear at face value to be rather odd. After all, we don't need to be genius to have anxiety. This is true but as proven in various clinical studies, you are more likely to experience clinical anxiety if you have a higher IQ. There are many reasons for this. Those with a higher IQ are more likely to overthink situations and have a higher level of self-awareness and those with higher IQs will over analyse and look for patterns and logic which are not always present in day-to day situations. Anxiety doesn't reduce your IQ but it does impact a person's ability to reach their potential and achieve accordingly. Autism can also impact reaching your potential, meaning that the collision of a high IQ and autism will create an ideal breeding ground for anxiety. As we discussed in the education chapter, Charlotte experienced a full range of academic levels when she was at school. In junior school, she was put in the year below, then went on to being average and eventually achieved high academic grades. Charlotte has an IQ of 181. This means that statistically, she is a genius. When she hears the word genius, she pictures a scientist or Albert Einstein. Looking simply at her IQ, Charlotte feels she has underachieved and this has caused her lots of anxiety over the years.

Danielle and Charlotte often discuss their sons' presentations. Both of their boys have diagnoses of anxiety disorders. However, these present very differently. There will be lots of reasons for this but we believe the primary reason for the difference lies in their cognitive ability. Kiddo is cognitively able. He has a talent for maths, knows the periodic table, and has a high level of IT ability. Pie has a diagnosed intellectual disability and despite being 9 years older than Kiddo, he is functioning at a much lower level.

Suppose we use the example of time. Kiddo is acutely aware of time; he can tell the time and he knows what time things should happen. He understands dates, days and their relationship with each other. Pie doesn't understand the concept of time. He has learnt some echolalic responses and phrases and might say, "in five minutes I will play" but that is nothing more than figurative speech. What has this all got to do with anxiety we hear you ask? Kiddo knows exactly when things should happen. Routine and structure underpin and scaffold his daily life. If something doesn't happen at the anticipated time, this is an instant anxiety trigger. He needs to understand why something hasn't happened and reassurance that it hasn't happened to try to keep his anxiety under control.

Pie doesn't have these anxieties as time is a concept his brain can't understand. The nearest he gets to understanding time is now and later. This means that if something happens five minutes late Pie won't be aware of that, meaning that it is an anxiety trigger he doesn't have to deal with.

Whilst there is a correlation between high IQ and the prevalence of clinical anxiety, it doesn't mean that those with a lower IQ are immune from anxiety at all. What it does mean is that how it presents, as well as interventions and treatments, are different.

Kiddo (along with Danielle and Charlotte) will at times be anxious about events that haven't yet happened or the idea of doing something. Most of Pie's anxieties are more predictable. He has had a lifetime of invasive medical treatment and the words "blood test" are a major anxiety trigger. He knows what a blood test is, he has had hundreds of them, and he has learnt through lived experience that he finds blood tests painful. He knows that often the result of the blood test leads to him needing more tests or a new treatment. This sort of known situation is always a trigger of anxiety for Pie.

When Pie was first accepted into Child Adolescent Mental Health Services (CAMHS), he was immediately medicated but also supported by a fantastic mental health nurse who was trained in Autism and Intellectual Disability. She worked with Pie for 3 years and gently tried a variety of holistic interventions. Pie couldn't engage in these despite his and their best efforts. His cognitive and emotional intelligence was too low. He was unable to rationalise or understand the triggers of his anxiety and if anything, the attempts at therapy caused him greater levels of anxiety as he became confused.

Regardless of IQ, there are still lots of ways that autism makes Pie more likely to be anxious. A lot of the anxiety triggers we talk about in this book are still relatable to an autistic child or young person with an intellectual disability. Not being able to find talking or play therapy to help Pie hasn't meant that we rely entirely on drug therapy to support his anxiety. There are still things that we can do to mitigate his anxiety and whilst these are not "official therapies" we have found that having a consistent approach amongst his entire care team helps enormously.

The difference in presentation between an autistic child with intellectual disabilities compared to an autistic child with a typical cognition level can make it more difficult to get help, or even get its causes acknowledged. If medication is prescribed, then it can be difficult to evaluate its effectiveness as there is a greater emphasis on the observations of others than the patient's voice.

There will be a variety of reasons why an individual has impaired cognition. The most common causes are genetic, congenital or brain injury which can impact a person's mental health regardless of external and/or environmental factors. They may also present with symptoms that could be attributed to either a psychiatric or neurological cause. These investigations take time and can delay treatment and interventions.

Whilst the everyday needs of an autistic child with an intellectual disability will be more far-reaching than an autistic child with typically functioning cognition as a general rule, we believe that anxiety has a more profound impact on the latter. Pie is almost 18. He will never live independently, never be able to work, and never manage his own money. His anxiety will be based on known situations and for most of his time he will be cocooned by those who love and understand him and a few trusted carers who have been selected and trained by us to ensure they can meet his needs in the familiar setting of his family home.

In contrast, when we were approaching 18, we were embarking on several 'A' Level examinations, preparing for university, and applying for student loans. We were breaking through from our cocoon and the anxious neurodivergent children were about to emerge into the world as anxious neurodivergent adults, which in the main were and have been disguised to the world as in control, capable and able adults. Whilst we are fortunate to be in this situation, it is important to remember that the exposure to anxiety triggers for autistic individuals in this category is so much greater and often unrelenting.

CHAPTER FIVE

Anxiety and Boundaries

"Autistic children don't like boundaries"

This myth is often promoted by parents and professionals alike but often this is not the case. This assumption is often made early in a child's life when the parent isn't even aware their child is autistic. They will be imposing neurotypical boundaries and delivering them in a neurotypical fashion. The outcome of this with a neurodivergent child is often explosive and leads parents to withdraw boundaries as, of course, all you want is to see your child happy and fulfilled. It's completely understandable.

This situation doesn't help the child or parent/professional as much as many would hope. The child can begin to struggle with simple daily demands, such as choosing a breakfast cereal. It's hard to understand why things have gone so wrong when all you wanted was for your child to be happy and feel they could be themselves. In this chapter, we explain how boundaries can be hugely positive for autistic children if they are implemented differently.

How do boundaries help reduce anxiety?

Boundaries are often portrayed as the root of all evil. Let's take the following scenario to demonstrate how a lack of boundaries can contribute to anxiety in autistic children.

In this daily routine, there are no structures or boundaries. The thermometer shows the level of stress an autistic child could experience when faced with too many choices and no boundaries.

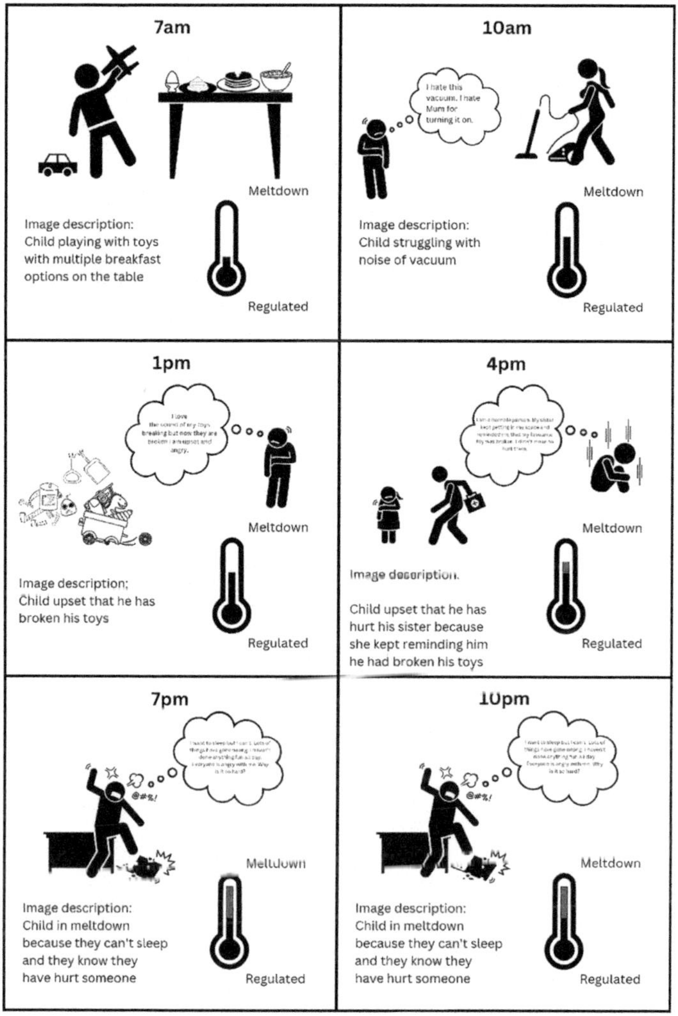
7am
Meltdown
Image description:
Child playing with toys with multiple breakfast options on the table
Regulated
10am
I hate this vacuum. I hate Mum for turning it on.
Meltdown
Image description:
Child struggling with noise of vacuum
Regulated
1pm
Meltdown
Image description;
Child upset that he has broken his toys
Regulated
4pm
Meltdown
Image description.
Child upset that he has hurt his sister because she kept reminding him he had broken his toys
Regulated
7pm
@#%!
Meltdown
Image description:
Child in meltdown because they can't sleep and they know they have hurt someone
Regulated
10pm
@#%!
Meltdown
Image description:
Child in meltdown because they can't sleep and they know they have hurt someone
Regulated

Now, let's take a look at a day with structure and more limited choices.

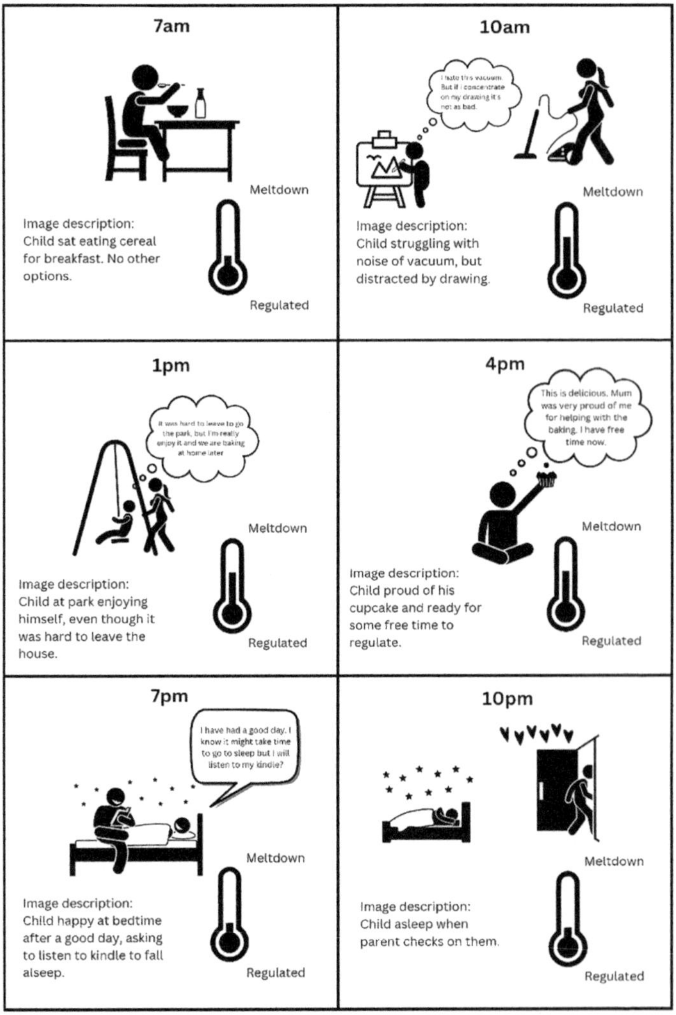

Whilst these examples are illustrative, and the reality will be somewhere in between, usually having a structure to the day helps. Charlotte knows if she wakes up and has no set points or structure, she can lose entire days. She ends up wandering around with no focus and not burning up enough energy, not just physical energy, but mental energy too. This means her brain starts questioning and going into overdrive. This overdrive can result in the spiralling of either impulsivity or questioning. Both are just as dangerous and impact her mental well-being.

How choices can make anxiety worse

Life is full of choices. Every day we make thousands of choices. Some are inconsequential, whilst others are life-changing. Learning to make a choice is an essential life skill. Making a choice allows us to develop as a person in our own right, and our decisions shape who we are as well as keep us safe. Charlotte can remember when Pie was 4. He used to attend a therapy group to improve his speech, language and motor skills. All the excellent work by this group was overshadowed by the constant offering of multiple choices to the four children who attended. Regardless of the communication difficulties they experienced (all were non-verbal), the children were overwhelmed by the choices.

The sessions started with a song about animals. During one session Pie was given a large poster with 20 pictures on it so he could select his animal. The result was shut down, leading to him never going back into the room again. A couple of weeks later, the occupational therapist asked what the problem was. She seemed genuinely shocked that Pie would have found that overwhelming and anxiety-inducing. I saw her a few years later and she was humble enough to confirm that on reflection (and more practice experience) she could see the mistakes and now used individual cards and gave limited choices geared to the individual child.

Limiting the number of choices is an important balance to ensure your child has their opinions heard and valued safely and securely. For children with ADHD in particular, rather than shut down because they have too many choices, they might impulsively choose without thinking. Having made their choice, they may then feel it is not the right one, which in turn causes anxiety as they have to do something they didn't want to.

Eradicating the impact that choices have on your child's anxiety is straightforward. It means:

- frequently reviewing your child's capacity to make choices
- deciding how many options you will give them
- how you are going to communicate the options
- how your child is going to communicate their decision.

Remember, verbal communication can be hard for verbal individuals as well as non-verbal ones. If your child is already anxious, reducing the number of options, as well as the number of choices within each option, is a simple way of offering effective support.

Discipline

A structure is a form of boundary, it encases the framework of the day or an allotted time. What happens when we are looking at behavioural boundaries though? This can be where things become tricky.

Often it needs to be evaluated closely. Consistency is key to success whilst being mindful of the bigger picture. Often, an autistic child's first experience of being disciplined will not have been dealt with correctly. One of the first times Charlotte remembers as a child was by a friend of her grandmother's. She said hello to Charlotte and Charlotte raised her hand in a wave. She was 5 and would only say a few words to caregivers. The friend told Charlotte she was "a rude little girl that needed to learn manners". Her grandmother, who was very insightful for someone born in 1917, responded with, "she was saying hello in her own way" and that Charlotte wasn't being rude. Despite her grandmother standing up for Charlotte, she remembers feeling angry, confused and resentful. This is a big problem with people who don't understand the needs of the child, wading in with their ideals of disciplining.

In contrast, Charlotte can remember the positive experiences of being disciplined. One example was when she was at primary school and she shouted "go away" at a child. They were wanting her to play with them. Charlotte didn't want to play or have them anywhere near her. Her loud outburst was not an expectation of the 1980s classroom, and she was hastily taken to the headteacher's office. The headteacher must have noticed her absolute shock that what she had done wasn't deemed acceptable. She explained to Charlotte that the child had been upset at being told to go away. She was equally quick to explain that Charlotte had done well to use her words to express what she needed. Putting a context around what Charlotte had done helped her.

This positive approach to discipline was essential. Charlotte couldn't read social cues or conventions. At the same time, her neurodivergent difference was just that and she would have to somehow learn to function in the alien environment known as "the world". We are not saying that being disciplined is always positive. What we do know is that when discipline is handled well, it is instrumental in enabling a child to function in a neurotypical world. Whilst there is an expectation and requirement for society to make reasonable adaptions and adjustments to enable autistic people to function, it is a two-way street.

The fear of not fitting in is massive for many autistic people, as is the fear of failure and being rejected. If you are not taught right from wrong or some idea of expected behaviours, you won't fit in and will be more likely to be rejected and underachieve.

Keeping those reasonable adjustments in mind, here are some things to consider when deciding when and how to discipline your child.

- Never discipline a child for having a meltdown, stimming or any other behaviour or communication which is genuinely out of their control.
- Use language appropriate to their developmental age. This might not even be the same at two points on the same day. It's dependent on the environment and how much they are having to process.
- Don't overuse words.
- Don't use punishments that can't or won't be followed through.
- Don't use punishments which involve the removal of items or strategies that are part of your child's regulation tool kit.
- Once the behaviour has stopped, reassure your child that they have now made the right choice.
- Don't bring up bad behaviour events that are in the past.
- Make sure they understand what they did was wrong and why. There is no point at all in simply telling a child, "stop that, it is naughty"

Remember, all children push boundaries at some point. All children have the right to be given the tools to keep safe and to be accepted.

CHAPTER SIX

Social Anxiety

The anxiety of social situations isn't only experienced by autistic people or those with ADHD. There will always be people with extravert or introvert personality preferences and both these psychological types (and everything in between) are open to presentations of anxiety around social situations. It's human nature and necessary to survive. The addition of autism often means there is already a predisposition to find social situations challenging.

The views of others

The behaviour of neurodivergent people means that they are more likely to be subjected to people commenting about them, especially during childhood. As a child, Charlotte remembers well people commenting on her not talking, not looking at them or fidgeting. These phrases can resound in your head and before you know it you are scared to be in a social situation. In Charlotte's case, it wasn't because she was remotely bothered by what other people thought of her, but rather that she was wondering what was being said about her when she wasn't there. This additional pressure means that there is an extra level of anxiety in simply accessing a social situation.

As well as commenting on social communication differences, a large challenge is when people feel it is their place to comment on behaviour. This is sadly the case in a lot of mainstream school playgrounds. Charlotte has seen first-hand the negative impact of a neurodivergent child being labelled as "the naughty one". This label will remain with that child and is in most cases an almost instant exclusion from social activities. If by some miracle "the naughty child" is included in any birthday parties or play dates, their behaviour will be under far more scrutiny than neurotypical children because there will be anticipation that something will happen.

Whilst none of us can control the views (however unfounded) of others on our child, or any other topic, the anxiety that these situations cause can be mitigated to some degree by advocating for your child. Charlotte can remember standing in the playground with her grandmother whilst a parent of another child commented on her lack of speech, eye contact and fidgeting. Even in the 1980s (when criticism of children from any adult was perceived as normal) her resourceful Grandmother would tell them what Charlotte's strengths were. All of us have a strength regardless of any difference or disability. Whilst advocating for your child, make the person understand why there may be certain presentations of behaviour, but at the same time make sure they know your child's strengths.

Relationships with other parents

As well as ensuring that the views of parents don't cause or worsen social anxiety for your child, the relationship that you have with other parents is also important. This is particularly true during the primary school years and can help your child develop some level of resilience to social situations and the anxiety they can trigger. Having a child with additional needs means that as parents we must spend so much of our time explaining to professionals what our children can't do, or what needs to be changed for an activity to be made accessible. There is no doubt about it, this can feel overwhelming and all-consuming. However, parents of typically developing children mustn't perceive you as the parent who is always complaining or moaning. Most parents moan about their children from time to time. Ensuring your child is perceived positively by other parents from what you say, will help give the child the best possible social experiences when they need them most, in their formative years.

Sensory impacts

Even in your own home, social situations may be a huge challenge. It's not uncommon to find social situations considerably more challenging at home, as changes cause a predictable environment to become unpredictable and in turn scary and negative. Therefore, you must be vigilant for potential triggers that may cause anxiety.

For example, if you know that your child struggles with hand driers in public bathrooms, they may relate going out of the house to hearing noisy hand driers. These would then need to be avoided. Otherwise, the picture created in your child's mind of going out will include that negative, overwhelming and anxiety-inducing sensory experience. Remember, the sensory impact of social situations is not only going to include items like hand driers. Charlotte struggles when she has additional people sitting in her living room. It looks different. Her motor planning is different to move around the room, as the entire visual map of the room has changed. This is where safe spaces are a go-to for reducing anxiety, as there is a space where your child can find a familiar, unchanged environment where they can regulate and be themselves. For more on how to create an effective safe space, visit our website https://www.autability.co.uk/safe-spaces

Visitor anxiety

This is a difficult one to balance. The visitor may be a close family member, friend or professional. They may be someone that your child likes or someone that your child wants to see. By contrast, they might be someone that they don't want to see. It doesn't overly matter what the personal views are of the visitor. It can be having another person in the house and the effort of having a visitor that is the problem. You have to communicate, and you will be expected to do certain things. This in itself is overwhelming. As an adult, this means we may not want to have any visitors. As a child or teen you don't often have control over this, so changing your household's attitude to visitors is essential to reduce anxiety. Following some of these ideas can help immensely:

- Be flexible. Make it clear to both child and visitor that there will not be an expectation for the child to see the visitor. This includes saying hello and goodbye.
- Keep it simple. Don't arrange a banquet and expect your child who normally eats a beige plate of food sat by themselves to suddenly sit down and eat different foods with different people.
- Keep it time-bound. This can be hard, but have a defined end time and stick to it. This means that there is a clear boundary around the entire visit which will help your child.
- Be prepared to cancel. Make sure that your guest is aware that this is a possibility that their visit may be cancelled at short notice.

The more your child trusts that these boundaries will be in place when it comes to visitors, the more accepting and less anxious they will be. Danielle went through a long period where no visitors at all were able to visit her family at home due to Kiddo's extreme anxiety, and his reactions when people came. Visitors caused him to self-injure due to distress, and he would constantly fear someone knocking on the front door. At one point it became so extreme that she had to put a sign up on the front door asking people not to knock or turn up unexpectedly. The constant anxiety meant Kiddo couldn't regulate himself at home, and this then affected his processing and ability to cope with simple everyday functioning. When Kiddo was able to understand, Danielle wrote a list of rules explaining that when someone came to visit Kiddo did not have to leave his room and that no one other than Mummy and Daddy would enter his room unless he gave permission. It was made clear to all visitors that children were NOT allowed upstairs at any time, even if they saw Kiddo sitting on the stairs watching them. If either Danielle or Kiddo's Dad had to spend the time during visits upstairs to supervise Kiddo, it was worth it in the long run. Kiddo became reassured that his bedroom was a safe space and trusted that no one would make him come downstairs. After many months of this, Kiddo began to edge further downstairs to see who was visiting. There was no pressure to say hello or even be verbal. The priority was giving him the confidence to be physically present in the same room as visitors, even if just for a moment.

Nowadays Kiddo can cope with one single visitor quite well. Danielle thinks this is due to his sensitivity around conversation and that with one visitor only, several conversations do not overlap due to multiple people talking, causing auditory overload. If they have multiple visitors, Kiddo can sometimes cope with being downstairs in a different room, but struggles to cope with multiple layers of conversation happening around him and can become distressed whilst demanding, "no talking!"

Kiddo will often say, "no one coming in!" so we know he can't cope with visitors. However, he can stay regulated and much calmer in the knowledge that he has his safe space whenever he needs it. If a delivery man knocks on the door, Kiddo will run upstairs at the speed of light! However, he feels safe in the knowledge no one will come into his room without his say-so, allowing him to remain relaxed in his own home.

Post Lockdown anxiety

The impact that the covid lockdowns had on social anxiety, and neurodivergent individuals in general, will be long-lasting. For months the message was, "outside is unsafe", and, "people outside of your household are not safe". This was followed by, "you can go out but keep your distance", and finally, "don't worry about covid". I imagine that these conflicting and changing statements are confusing enough for a neurotypical brain. The rigidity of thought experienced by autistic people means that these statements are even harder to justify and process. How can such serious messages suddenly overnight mean absolutely nothing? Or, suddenly become so serious you can't leave the house?

This means that in essence, our brains had to adapt to a new perception of what was safe outside, and having done this once we then had to adapt to various changes including the final one of, "everything is safe". This was not easy, especially as for such a long time we had also lost the skills of going out, being sociable etc. When we are in a routine, neurodivergent individuals can hold on to skills far more easily, as they are constantly practised. Just like learning to play an instrument, if you suddenly stop and don't have any lessons or practice for 3 months, you will find it much harder to pick up your instrument and start playing than if you had been continuously practising the entire time.

Danielle remembers finding reintegrating into the world post-lockdown extremely difficult. "How did I used to just come to the supermarket and buy things?" "What do I say to the checkout assistant, do we talk or not?" Such simple communication skills were forgotten, even as an adult in her late thirties who could talk continuously for hours on subjects of her choosing. Basic social interaction skills were no longer at the forefront of her mind, and this made going out a very mentally exhausting chore. Pre-planning what conversations may need to take place depending on her intended destination, and running through simple sequences such as purchasing goods or making bookings in her head before she went out was exhausting. There were times when she was too tired to leave the house by the time she felt prepared enough.

Now the world is open again, all those necessary skills are at the forefront of Danielle's mind, frequently used and active meaning that rehearsal isn't needed for everyday tasks and conversations.

It's not that Danielle would be silent if another person spoke to her after the lockdowns had finished. It was the fact she would stutter, say the wrong thing and frequently embarrass herself by saying something that was perceived as strange by other people. The anxiety of this happening was something she had to work through and is a primary reason she tries as much as possible to keep Kiddo going out into the outside world when she can. Starting again in terms of social skills can be extremely challenging.

Young neurodivergent children who experienced lockdown, along with their peers, have missed out on social developmental building blocks. This is hard enough for typically developing children but for neurodivergent children who already have impairment in social communication, the impact is far greater. Not only are these children having to re-process what is safe, but they are also having to relearn how to be sociable, what the outside world is and all whilst having missed out on a developmental stage.

News anxiety

Pie loves watching the news and so did Charlotte whilst growing up. She thinks there is something very appealing to some autistic brains about the familiarity of the presentation and factual elements of the news. It does however cause a lot of anxiety, especially if the entire story is not understood. Charlotte remembers growing up in London in the 1990s when there were regular terrorist alerts and a campaign of vigilance surrounding bins in public places. At the same time, there was the "Keep Britain Tidy" campaign. Charlotte found it impossible to process the bin as both a potential security threat and a good thing. She would try to avoid bins, crossing roads and looking out for them obsessively. She never put rubbish in a public bin, instead filling up her pockets and bags with litter.

It is important to know what is going on in the world and both Charlotte and Danielle will always watch the news. It is equally important to watch out for articles that could cause anxiety and have an open discussion with your child if necessary. Whilst we can't live in denial of the dangers we could face, there is a point where the awareness stops being healthy and becomes too much to process causing considerable anxiety.

Fashion anxiety

Even if an autistic person isn't sociable and isn't concerned about being accepted into a social group, it does not mean they are ok with standing out from the crowd. It isn't just a simple matter of finding the right clothing to 'fit in', our sensory processing impacts a lot of autistic people's ability to comfortably wear certain items of clothing. We must train our brains to find clothes we are comfortable wearing, with how they look and how they feel.

Danielle will forever be grateful to The Spice Girls for helping her survive her teenage years. Sporty Spice made comfortable exercise clothing fashionable, and there was a wave of various tracksuit bottoms and tracksuits being the latest trend. Whilst it didn't help on every occasion, she knew she could comfortably wear tracksuit bottoms, trainers and a name-brand t-shirt in most places whilst not sticking out like a sore thumb.

Working out what items of clothing we want to wear takes a great deal of executive functioning power, which can also reduce our threshold to becoming anxious. Even if you have a wardrobe full of clothing you are happy with it, choosing an outfit can be a massive task. Working out what you are going to wear for a particular occasion is a massive process which can take weeks. It can become all-consuming to the point that the anxiety over what to wear is so extreme that you end up not going out.

On many occasions, anxiety over clothing has caused Danielle to have extreme anxiety attacks before large social events and she has not been able to attend. The one event where she felt no stress about what she was going to wear in the slightest, was her wedding day. Now most of us are used to the image of a panicking bride, concerned that their dress isn't quite right or what people would think of it. Nope, Danielle knew that as long as she turned up in a white dress from a wedding dress shop, she couldn't fail. No matter what anyone's opinion of her dress was, she would be wearing the socially expected and acceptable attire for the occasion. Similarly when she has been asked to be a bridesmaid, the relief of not having to choose an outfit for the occasion has been huge. It wouldn't matter if she was dressed in a bin bag, she would be socially accepted because that would be what the bride wanted. So don't assume anxiety is all about being the centre of attention when it comes to fashion, sometimes being the centre of attention can take all the anxiety surrounding clothing away as the rules of what you should wear are so clear.

Who is coming?

For a lot of people, going to meet a friend and finding out on arriving that another person is with them who you weren't expecting isn't a big deal. For a lot of autistic people, this can be a complete disaster. It isn't down to who that extra person is (although that can have a huge impact), it is about the predicted picture of the event you thought you were attending being changed. Charlotte always remembers as a teenager, arranging to meet a friend from school at the swimming pool. When she arrived, they had invited another friend. Charlotte went into shutdown. The entire trip was wrong. She liked the other person present, but they were not supposed to be there. Even now if Charlotte goes swimming, she is still triggered by that one event from over 30 years ago. Nothing terrible happened, nobody said anything unkind or didn't include her, but the sudden change was something her brain couldn't process. Charlotte will still panic even now if she was meeting a friend, that someone else will be there that she was not expecting.

Danielle struggles in the same way and has had many times where she has been invited over to people's houses only to discover several other people were also visiting. The anxiety of this stopped her from socialising with some of her friends for a while. The worry of what to expect simply became too much and she would make excuses and cancel. For Danielle, the major issue is socialising in larger groups. The different personalities of people, different topics of conversation and changing her persona from person to person when there was more than just her and one other friend was exhausting. She could prepare for this if she knew exactly who was going, or if she knew there were going to be a large number of people she didn't know. But, if caught off guard, the whole experience was gut-wrenching. It would leave her longing for home.

So, if your kids are heading out and some extra people turn up, don't disregard it as minor. It could be a big deal to them.

Out-of-context anxiety

Many autistic people categorise others according to the environment where they usually see them. For example, your child will expect to see their teacher in school and not at the local supermarket. The same as unexpected visitors, meeting people out of their normal context is difficult to process and can be a real worry. It is something that can get resolved but can also take time to process.

Kiddo struggles with seeing children he knows from school at other locations. It causes him to panic. There are several reasons behind this panic, including the following:

- The people may look different. They will probably be wearing different clothes, which changes the way their face looks and their overall appearance to the picture he holds of them in his head.

- They may talk differently from what he is used to. Maybe they feel safer expressing their emotions around family or use words that only family know the meaning of.
- In a different environment, he has lost his cues. When Kiddo walks into the school reception in the morning, he follows a set pattern of actions and speech. For example, he might say, "Good morning!" and give the receptionist a high five. He sees the door and knows when he goes through it who he will see. He knows where he will walk, who he is likely to see and how the reception feels. The door reminds him he needs to say good morning, the corridor reminds him who is sitting in the office at the end of it and what their name is. All these environmental cues make it easy for his brain to work out what to say and how to behave. In a different environment, he doesn't have those predictable cues that jog his memory on the right things to say and the right actions to make, all of which have a track record of being safe. He might freeze when he sees a person out of context, wondering if 'good morning' is the right phrase because maybe it's the afternoon. Danielle has come across as very rude to people she has met out of context in the past, simply because she wasn't prepared to see them and didn't have immediate access to the information she needed about them at the forefront of her mind.

This might seem like a small issue and something that can be easily dealt with. It can be, but it is important not to dismiss the worry an autistic child may have. It's important to gradually explain how and why that person can be valued in more than one context. It isn't their appearance or the people they are with that make them who they are. The person seen out of context is still the same core person. It's just a few adjustments that need to be made to that picture of them which is held inside your child's head.

There will always be very individual and personal reasons for feeling anxiety around social activities. The good thing is that there are lots that you can do to support your child in this area once you can understand the root of the problem. Taking a supportive and non-judgemental approach is always key so that your child feels supported to take the next steps in trying to overcome their anxiety. As with all journeys of recovery, working slowly and steadily is essential. They don't want to feel pressured but at the same time, encouragement and a can-do attitude are the way forward. Charlotte was recently working with a young person who hadn't been to a shop for a long time. He was terrified, but he did it. When his mum asked him how he felt afterwards he said, "I felt sick at the time, but now I feel great!"

CHAPTER SEVEN

The importance of educating yourself

This will be one of the few times when you read the word 'education' in one of our books, and we won't be referring to that oh-so-familiar battle to secure your child the correct education package. What we mean is the importance of education and knowledge so you can support your child's anxiety and mental health. Often, the need for parental education is mentioned to parents in the wrong way, at the wrong time and it goes something like this:

Parent: "I am struggling with my child's development"

Professional: "I will send you to a parenting class"

All this does is reaffirm the parent's insecurity that they are somehow to blame for the challenges their child is facing. What is being offered is not a parenting course, it is education on how to support a child or young person with a specific difference or disability.

Sometimes these "parenting classes" are offered as a prerequisite to a child being offered any other form of support or intervention. This is never a solution, especially in a situation when all that does is put the already exhausted parent under even more pressure, with added guilt that if they don't manage to go that their child won't be given the treatment that they so desperately need. Over the years Charlotte and Danielle have attended and declined these opportunities in equal measure for a variety of reasons. Charlotte remembers soon after Pie's autism diagnosis, attending an "about autism" course for parents. It was run by two very enthusiastic ladies, but their knowledge did not match their enthusiasm. Even then, with Charlotte's much more limited knowledge of parenting an autistic child, she knew that there were inaccuracies in what was being said. It did however encourage her to read books about autism. She opted for a combination of books aimed at parents and professionals. At the time, most books aimed at parents were autobiographical accounts which whilst interesting had very little relevance to her son's presentation.

On the day of Kiddo's diagnosis, Danielle was told not to attend the course the NHS would usually recommend as she knew too much. However, Danielle's knowledge was far less than Charlotte's. Danielle had also read books containing both practical advice and personal stories in the lead-up to Kiddo's assessment, which helped. Both experienced such a different approach to "parenting courses".

Over the years Charlotte has learnt that the best way forward is to accept any form of information and advice which is offered, filter it and work out what is relevant to your child. Sometimes, information that isn't relevant at the time you receive it can become useful at a point in the future.

Supporting your child's anxiety is no different and by reading this guide you have already committed to educating yourself to support your child. However, education needs to go further. It is about educating others, not about autism and anxiety but about how autism and anxiety impact your child's daily life. There is a subtle difference, and you are one of the only people that can do that. Let's take the example of your child becoming anxious at the prospect of visitors because they don't want to have to talk to the guests until they are ready. Your role is to explain this to the guests before they arrive. Whilst this may not mitigate your child's anxiety instantly, over time they realise that this stress has been removed. This allows them to relax a bit and then they will make progress.

The same is true of any professional or person that comes into regular contact with your child. Educating yourself doesn't only allow you to advocate for your child more effectively, but if you can identify triggers for your child then you can reduce them. If your child is struggling to access something they enjoy, for example, bowling, because it is busy and too frantic, find out what time is quieter and go then. The first time you may only just go to the premises to show your child that it is quiet and build it up as their anxiety reduces.

Even the most educated parent will not have all the answers and the journey in supporting your autistic's child anxiety will not always be smooth. However, armed with the accurate and relevant information you will be as prepared as possible.

How to arm yourself with the right knowledge to help your child

We've talked about the importance of educating yourself, but what does this mean in practical terms? Here are a few ways you can make sure you've got adequate knowledge about a venue, event or visit that may help alleviate some stress in your anxious child.

- *Visit venues to familiarise yourself with the layout*

You can do this by yourself or with your child, whichever works better for them. If your child doesn't want a pre-visit, take photos or a video as you walk in. Include key places of interest such as toilets, where to get food and drink and a meeting place in the event they want to leave early and get away from other people.

- *Double-check with venues if there are any special events on*

Special events at venues can change lighting, noise, entry points and much more. There is no point doing a pre-visit to a venue if it's going to look and feel completely different on the day your child is going. So, double-check with the manager or check online. There's nothing worse than going to all this effort than to find out on the day it meant nothing.

- *Ask hosts about schedules and details*

Some events will be held at people's homes or purpose-built venues such as a marquee. If you think having information about the party/wedding/reception or meal would help alleviate anxiety levels then do not feel embarrassed about asking the host for details. It may be that they don't know the details yet, in which case explain why you are asking (see next section). Maybe they could pop the details in an email or text so your child can read them. If you do this, it's essential to explain the importance of sticking to the plan they send at the event itself, so that your child's anxiety isn't triggered.

- *Length of stay*

Whether you're going to visit someone else or they're coming to visit you, talk timescales. It may be that your child can tolerate people in your home if they know exactly when they will be leaving. This gives them control over when they come down, how much they talk to visitors and if they decide not to come down at all, how long they will need to stay in another room.

- *Guestlist*

Finding out who is going can relieve a tonne of anxiety. It helps you plan conversation, process what to dress and prepare how you want to present yourself. Whilst masking isn't always healthy, it is a common survival technique and many may choose to use it so that they can start to overcome their anxiety. So, find out who is going to be there.

All these things can help alleviate some anxiety and all are easily achieved by educating yourself on a situation or event.

Practical ways to educate others

As well as educating yourself you must educate others. This doesn't mean you should only inform people of what makes your child anxious, but also about things that don't. Being asked to take part in projects, do jobs or help out in ways that don't increase anxiety are huge confidence boosters to a child. They are key to recovery, so don't forget them!

There are several simple ways you can educate others about your child's anxiety:

- *Inform people with plenty of notice*

Warning people your child might be anxious can help immensely. That being said, in some cases people knowing about a child's fears can make children more anxious. If you can, then ask your child which they would prefer. If your child isn't able to engage in that conversation then you can make an educated decision. Whatever you do, do not go against any clear wishes your child has made for how to handle a situation. Doing so could cause a huge breakdown in trust and further setbacks. Trust in others is key when it comes to recovery from anxiety.

- *Provide written information sheets*

In formal environments, such as schools and hospitals, having information in writing on record that staff members can refer to can be crucial. This doesn't need to be an essay on the life history of your child. Staff are busy and need key facts that are easy to reach at a moment's notice. To see examples of how to present such information, see our 'All About Me Forms' here.

- *Be reasonable*

Having suffered from GAD since she was 17, Danielle knows there are often a million and one things that can be done to alleviate a person's anxiety. However, that doesn't mean you should expect them all to be done. Being reasonable is what will get you listened to. Concentrate on the core triggers and explain there might be more but you know it's not always possible to remember all the information, especially when a class of 30 children are involved. The child needs enough support to access the activity and this will help them build their resilience. It can be a tough road for them, but it will help them as they grow to start understanding how they can help themselves, as well as using the support from others.

Remember, you are the chief educator on how to ease your child's anxiety. Be discrete, do it in writing, and not in front of the child unless the child wants to educate someone themselves. This is something to be hugely encouraged only when they are ready and shows acceptance of their condition as well as an understanding of it.

CHAPTER EIGHT

Autism, anxiety and sleep

Sleep. For a parent of an autistic child, it is often known as a legend. Some mythical state that most people seem to enjoy but for you, it is rarer than gold. You struggle to get your child to fall asleep, stay asleep, want sleep, anything to do with sleep can seem like a real challenge most of the time. Throw in some anxiety (they don't have to have received a formal diagnosis) and you've got yourself a conundrum. Sleep feels so far away you wonder if your child will ever reach it. In this chapter, we will talk about whether autism, anxiety, or both are potentially the cause of your child's sleep problems, and what you can do to give you all the best chance possible at getting some shut-eye.

Autism and sleep

For some autistic children, sleep difficulties may be purely down to a predisposition linked to their autism. Others may have a separate sleep condition though, and this can take a long time to work out.

To neurotypical people, situations that make them feel a bit on edge are perceived as everyday events. For autistic people, they can be massive. This isn't because they are prone to exaggeration, but because their brain simply can't work everyday situations out. You might hear professionals talk about autism causing anxiety. This is usually what is meant by that. By simply being a minority in this world, things will always be just that little (or huge) bit more difficult. This is where the processing comes in, and why processing time is so essential during the day.

Without quiet time to reflect and process the events of the day during the daytime itself, you're left thinking through everything at the first opportunity you are given which is often bedtime. And sometimes, even with processing time during the day, you are still left thinking everything through when you lay down to sleep at night.

Sometimes conversations, events or interactions become all-encompassing and until you have worked out what they mean, you are left searching for every pattern, every piece of logic and every way to understand what has happened. So don't think a handy two-hour downtime period after school is going to sort out the sleep problem. It will most likely help, but the role of being autistic in having sleep difficulties is far more complex than that.

Once sleep hasn't happened a couple of times, you then have the added complication of a routine that you don't want. The rigidity of thought and the expectation that things reoccur in a pattern means that very quickly there is an inner expectation that sleep won't happen. Again, this isn't about being dramatic or making up a self-fulfilling prophecy, it's just the way we process the world and strangely, knowing you won't sleep is almost a comfort because it is expected.

There is also the impact of sensory processing on sleep. This can be the need for deep pressure or the need for sensory input. Most parents will have a vision of their child sleeping in a dark quiet room. In reality, your child may need the complete opposite. Some autistic people need several sensory stimuli such as lights on or background noise. This may be hard to do as it goes against what people think is needed to support their child's sleeping habits. For more on this, see our chapter on sleep in 'Parenting Rewired'.

Anxiety and sleep

Anxiety is known to have a detrimental impact on sleep. Anxious people are also more likely to have vivid dreams and nightmares. As a result, the child or young person can then become anxious about falling asleep for fear of experiencing vivid dreams.

People with clinical anxiety often have higher levels of adrenaline meaning that their body is constantly in "fight or flight" mode. This means your brain is continually judging whether you should run from or fight any threat that approaches you. Now you might be thinking, "no threat is going to approach my child at home?" with visions of an angry lion bounding in through your front door. That's the level of event that SHOULD evoke a fight or flight response. When you are overly anxious, something so small as the sound of a tap dripping can give you that same response that you would experience when an angry lion does come charging through your front door. In short, you're way over-sensitive and treating non-threats as actual life-threatening events, which is not conducive to a good night's sleep (understatement). Your brain is on high alert and even if your body is exhausted, your brain will not change down a gear owing to the impact of the higher adrenaline levels.

Once this happens, not only do you have the problem of not being able to fall asleep, but you begin to worry about the events of that day, what is happening tomorrow and in fact, anything. These thoughts in turn increase brain activity, making sleep even more unlikely.

The challenge of falling asleep

An autistic person with anxiety may find falling asleep hugely difficult. To sleep, you have to be able to relax enough, and this is where being neurodivergent and having anxiety can hit your sleep. As previously mentioned, autistic people often take longer to process daily events, conversations and feelings. During the evenings, many children are expected to socialise with their family, talk at the dinner table and do homework. None of this allows for quality processing time, so if your child doesn't have this downtime after school, introduce it now. They may need to play video games, listen to music or draw. Don't assume because they're doing an activity that they aren't processing. We all process differently and some of us (particularly those with ADHD) need to occupy one part of our mind so we can process with another.

So, if you're autistic, and don't have your processing needs met, most of the time you can forget sleep. But what about if you suffer from anxiety as well? Anxiety, as we know, is a fear of the future. A fear of things to come. Being autistic can mean wanting to plan for every eventuality so that you will know what to do and how to act when amongst neurotypicals. If your autistic child is anxious about school, an event or even a conversation they know they need to have, you can effectively double the amount of processing it would take a neurotypical person. That is one active brain, and an active brain isn't going to relax and fall asleep easily.

If eventually, they do manage to fall asleep (and it can take hours), this is because their brain has slowed down for long enough to allow sleep to finally take over. We must remember though, that many autistic people require less sleep than neurotypicals. Trying to make an autistic child fall asleep too early for their brain simply will not work. After processing time, they may not be tired for a while. So, pick a time to send your child to bed when they are showing genuine signs of tiredness such as yawning and sleepy eyes. It may seem mad to send your 6-year-old to bed at 11 pm, but maybe that's just what they need.

What if you fall asleep, but wake up in the night?

But what about those who fall asleep easily but wake up constantly in the night? If you're suffering from anxiety, it's likely your brain won't relax during sleep as much as it should. We've all had those nights where we have been asleep, but we don't feel like we have slept. This is because (in very basic terms) your brain hasn't relaxed enough and has still been working to some extent.

Many feel the key to helping an anxious person sleep lies in what we do at night time. We picture lavender pillows, sounds of waves breaking on the shores etc. Whilst these soothing methods can be very effective, they're going to mean diddly squat if your child's anxiety and processing haven't been cared for during the day. So many sleep problems relating to anxiety are fixed by dealing with the anxiety that we experience during the day. Many do not realise this and place all their efforts into relaxing evenings or sleep medication. They might help, and they might even work, but one thing is for sure – they will not cure your autistic anxious child's sleep problem.

At this point, it's important to consider whether it's anxiety or being autistic and/or ADHD that is causing sleep problems. How you attempt to improve your child's sleep will hugely depend on this. If it's both, then you might have double your work cut out, but don't worry as hopefully, we can help you.

Autism, anxiety and lack of sleep

So, if being autistic can make you more prone to being anxious simply by having to live and get by in this world, it's often likely that sleep problems are a combination of both. How can you tell whether autism, anxiety or a combination of both, are the main reason your child is struggling with sleep?

For some, there will be a change in behaviour that makes this obvious. Kiddo slept until he was about 18 months old. Then BAM. Overnight he stopped. Shock to the system didn't even cover it, it was such a huge behaviour change. It started when Danielle took him on their very first holiday. A change of room, a change of bed, a change of bathroom before bed. All of it was way too much for Kiddo to process, and he couldn't fall asleep until gone 2 am. Thinking it was just a blip, Danielle was sure sleep would return when they came home. Nope. That. Was. It. Sleep was a distant memory. Kiddo took a minimum of 3 hours to fall asleep, often longer. BUT (and this is a big but), he was happy. He would chat away to himself, fidget, play with his toys etc. Yes, there was the typical raging "I'm not tired!" scream, but as a parent, you ignore that and think they will fall asleep soon enough because they were tired.

Kiddo had other ideas.

Danielle didn't want to be sat in his room until he fell asleep, but Kiddo started to become agitated if she wasn't there. Not wanting bedtime to become a scream fest, she would sit on the landing with part of her foot showing where Kiddo could see it. It might sound bonkers, but it worked and was enough to keep him settled until eventually, he entered the land of nod. The evenings became lost to Danielle and her routine was suddenly sitting on the landing for several hours a night whilst he fell asleep. She got it down to fine art in the end. Books, snacks, Kiddo's Dad would bring dinner up to the landing etc. It was a well-known routine with her friends because she was messaging them all evening. Talking out loud to Kiddo's Dad only made Kiddo want to get up more.

This may sound like an awful lot of fuss, and it was. At the time though, they didn't know Kiddo was autistic and thought this was just some terrible twos phase that he would grow out of. It was only when they visited a paediatrician that they realised it wasn't. It was clear that whatever was happening, it wasn't 'typical' development.

Enter, melatonin. Melatonin was a life changer for Danielle. Kiddo went from three hours plus drop-off time to twenty minutes. Incredible! She had her evenings back with her husband. Blissfully unaware of what problems melatonin would create, they had maybe two evenings where they stayed up late watching TV. And then, it started.

The midnight wake-ups. Melatonin can be wonderful at getting you off to sleep. However, it doesn't keep you asleep and once this kid was up, he was up. Some nights he slept until 2 am, but 99% of the time, Kiddo woke between midnight and 1.30 am. The melatonin had helped him drop off beautifully, but the fact was that he still had a very active brain that was processing EVERYTHING. This was autism-based sleep difficulties at its finest, with some ADHD thrown in.

Every idea under the sun was tried to get Kiddo some shut-eye. In the end, Danielle got a referral to a London-based hospital to seek the advice of a sleep specialist. They explained all about how melatonin works and in Kiddo's case, some more medication was prescribed to try and keep him asleep a bit longer. What was evident is that the lack of sleep was impacting Kiddo's daily life and although he couldn't sleep, he needed to. Some autistic people don't seem to need as much sleep, but the research on that is ongoing.

Although Kiddo was happy, the consultant said something that Danielle won't ever forget.

"You are quite possibly going to need help with anxiety given his neurodevelopmental profile, and I'd recommend you do that soon so it doesn't become another impact on his sleep".

Sure enough, 4 years later when Kiddo was 7/8 years old, the sleep difficulties took a huge change in direction.

Enter lockdown. The most peculiar time for autistic people. On the one hand, it was an amazing break from face-to-face socialising on a large scale, but on the other hand, when it came to an end, many of us had lost the skills we had for coping in the outside world. Anxiety levels rose hugely, and this is when Kiddo's sleep got worse again but in a completely different way.

He went from being happy before bed to becoming extremely stressed at the thought of sleep. Not because of the sleep itself, but because sleep meant the arrival of tomorrow and that was a thought he couldn't tolerate at all. Phrases such as "no sleep!" and "no tomorrow!" would ring out through the house at high volume. He refused to go to his bedroom and when he did eventually give in and go, a parent had to be with him at all times. At the absolute peak of his anxiety, he would find ways to keep himself awake until 5 am or later, because in his mind if he didn't sleep, then tomorrow wouldn't arrive.

Even the realisation that nothing could stop tomorrow wasn't enough to make him give in to sleep. Staying awake slowed time down for him. He didn't close his eyes and suddenly wake up with no warning. He could prepare, count down the hours, and then the arrival of the morning was no longer such a shock. Kiddo was so anxious that he did ANYTHING to stop himself from sleeping. When either parent tried to remove what he was using to keep himself awake, the distress was so extreme that there was even less chance of him sleeping. There had to be a compromise.

The example of Kiddo's change in behaviour regarding sleep is a dramatic one. His autistic profile plays a huge part in this. Many children and young people may quietly stay awake in bed worrying about tomorrow or the day after. They may be able to talk it through with parents or caregivers, which could be a major help in processing. When Danielle was a teenager, many nights her Mum would find her awake late into the night. Sometimes it was something so small and easily fixed, such as worrying about what clothes she was going to wear the next day. From then on, she always laid her clothes out the night before and asked her mum to help make decisions between items if she was too anxious to do so.

Making sure it's not something which is easily remedied is often a missed trick. To neurotypicals, not knowing what you are going to wear the next day may not seem anxiety-provoking in the slightest. To an autistic person though, when there is so much to process and so many transitions to navigate, the brain is so busy that seemingly small decisions can be quite big ones due to decision fatigue and general exhaustion from processing. This makes sleep even more essential for the brain to recover each night. So, whilst with Kiddo the change to anxiety being the primary cause of no sleep was obvious, this may not always be the case.

In some people, certain sleep patterns become so ingrained that they can be difficult to break. Even when everything is OK and anxiety is low, the brain may be so used to waking at a certain time that it will continue to do so. Danielle had years of Kiddo waking between midnight and 2 am. After many years of trying different medications and sleep techniques, eventually, they were able to improve his sleep. However, Danielle still wakes at 2 am every single night. How successful she is at returning to sleep quickly depends on her anxiety levels. Through months of practice and essentially trying to train her brain, there are now nights that Danielle can return to sleep within 20 minutes of waking. But, bring in any anxiety or stress (of which there is a LOT being a parent carer) and she knows staying in bed and attempting to fall back asleep is futile. Racing thoughts and worries make it almost impossible.

In desperation, she started trying a few different things and eventually designed her reset routine. Danielle can tell within a few minutes whether her mind is relaxed enough to drift back off without getting out of bed. When it isn't, she gets up. She moves to another room, maybe has a small snack and a drink and plays games on her phone. These games don't require high intellectual effort, but just enough focus that her attention is taken away from her anxious thoughts. Sometimes she falls asleep where she is sitting, but usually, she can feel when her mind and body are ready for sleep again. She heads back to bed and is asleep within 20 minutes.

It can be hugely tempting to remove all electronics when encouraging sleep, and for the majority of people that is the best thing to do. Having an active anxious brain though requires taming and calming. Sometimes, watching that film you know every word to or playing that mindless game on your phone is what is needed to draw the focus away from what is stopping you sleep. There is, however, one thing to be wary of.

Kiddo started using his iPad to help him calm down at night when he was at the peak of his anxiety and worked brilliantly for about a week. He fell asleep listening to music and watching programmes he was familiar with. One night though there was a big difference, he was using his iPad to keep himself awake. That fear of sleep and tomorrow coming too quickly and without warning became so great, that he used the iPad to keep his brain working. He suddenly wasn't watching programmes or listening to music, he was building in his games. Whilst some will find that an excellent way to calm, for Kiddo it was stimulating, and he knew it. So did Danielle. In this instance, the iPad was removed (despite Kiddo's distress) and replaced with a speaker so he could still listen to his music and programmes. The aim was of course not to distress him, and his parents were aware that he still required comfort to ease any distress. A quiet dark room would not have sufficed, but sleep was still the aim and after 2 nights Kiddo was back to falling asleep at some point rather than staying awake for 24 hours.

It can be hard for parents, but sleep is a major health issue and sometimes tough decisions need to be made so that your child doesn't make their anxiety worse through lack of sleep.

Getting help

Not everyone is understanding, sadly. At this point, this is where evidence is required. Start keeping a sleep diary. This will show any patterns that perhaps link to poor sleep before or after a certain day or event. Nowadays you can get cheap watches that track sleep, and although they may not be necessarily as accurate as a device provided by a sleep clinic, they will at least give you data to show that there is a problem. Good old-fashioned sleep diaries are often enough, any factual evidence you can provide will help you make your case. You can't expect professionals to listen to how tired you are without providing some timing or evidence because people experience sleep differently. Take that data to your GP, school nurse, teacher, anyone. If the lack of sleep is becoming a major problem, then do take it up with your GP.

For a free sleep diary template, visit our website here https://www.autability.co.uk/product-page/sleep-diary

CHAPTER NINE

Pathological Demand Avoidance

Anyone who works with autistic children and their families will most likely have been made aware of Pathological Demand Avoidance (PDA) at some point. Some parents will say that their child has a diagnosis of PDA whilst others will describe it as PDA type ASD, or a PDA profile and various other descriptions. There is much confusion surrounding where PDA sits within autism, whether indeed it exists at all and what PDA is.

When a diagnosis is made there will be set out criteria which must be met for that diagnosis to be made. One of the greatest challenges when diagnosing something for which there is no biological test is that the clinician must rely on observations made by themselves and others. There are of course diagnostic manuals which set out the criteria that need to be met for a diagnosis to be made. The two main diagnostic manuals for such disorders are DSM-5 and ICD-10. Worldwide these manuals are referred to by medics when assessing patients and researching solutions to help them. Such guidelines help with understanding conditions and help to create awareness. In theory, they bring consistency to the assessment and diagnostic process, which is essential.

PDA has been recognised more in recent years, although it is not a new concept. PDA was first proposed as a syndrome by British child psychiatrist Elizabeth Newson in 1980. Newson has spent her career researching PDA and creating diagnostic criteria, but to date, this has not been officially accepted. It is widely believed that PDA is a trait of ASD, however, Newson sees PDA as a separate standalone syndrome. By contrast, PDA is mentioned by NICE in appendix 3 of their guidance on the assessment of autism as a trait or characteristic of ASD, but not as a standalone condition. The other challenge when looking at where PDA sits alongside autism is the ever-changing assessment criteria of autism. At the time when Newson was investigating her vision of PDA, the criteria for autism were very different to the diagnostic criteria found today in DSM-5 or ICD-10.

No wonder there is so much confusion surrounding PDA when there is no official or accepted guidance on what PDA is. Working with families who have autistic children we are often asked about Pathological Demand Avoidance or see it mentioned in feedback or comments on our posts. PDA is not mentioned as a condition in either DSM-5 or ICD-10 which means that there is not a uniform acknowledgement at this time of the existence of PDA or a clear assessment or diagnostic criteria.

Despite questions around the presentation, diagnostic criteria and the existence of PDA, there are a growing number of parents who are eager for acceptance of their child's PDA and a belief that individuals with a PDA profile need separate resources, along with an ever-growing desire from parents for acknowledgement.

We have heard families complain that PDA isn't diagnosed at their hospital, or that their local authority won't acknowledge it on their child's EHC plan. In contrast, we hear parents talk about their "relief" at receiving a PDA diagnosis and proudly parade it around like a peacock showing off their feathers knowing that they have managed to achieve something that others are saying is impossible.

With little official information on parenting children with SEND, there is a trend to get support from other parents in a similar situation, especially through social media channels. This kind of support can be useful and feel like a lifeline in your darkest hour. It can be great for signposting and general advice and support, but it can also be very detrimental. This is particularly true when dealing with unrecognised presentations such as PDA. As they can't be officially diagnosed, parents can easily be swept up into another parent(s) confusion and/or misunderstanding of how to support and help their child.

The same is happening with PDA. There is a high level of misunderstanding among parents and professionals, and this is exasperated by the lack of a clear diagnostic profile, assessment procedures and how to support these individuals in the longer term. All children avoid demands and will go through stages where this will appear almost constant, and reactions will be atypical and out of context. There is also the 'whisper' effect when parents pick up certain points and run with them. This is dangerous for everyone. It means that those who generally need help are sidelined or overlooked simply because of the numbers needing support. Some parents believe that putting demands on an autistic child is wrong and that creates more problems. There then comes a return to the blame of the parent culture in autism which started in the 1960s with the refrigerator mother syndrome and there is no progress at all in the understanding, acceptance and support for neurodivergent individuals.

There will also be those who argue that PDA can't be linked to autism because it wasn't seen previously. This argument returns us to the problems surrounding the changing profile of autism. In the 1980s a person with an autism diagnosis would have most likely attended a special needs school and then lived in a residential care home. There would have been limited demands on these individuals as they were sidelined by society and would have had limited demands and expectations put on them.

Two major changes since then are the much-welcomed understanding and inclusion of disabled people, meaning that they are now valued members of society and their gifts and talents are recognised. The second change is the change from autism to a broader diagnosis of autism spectrum disorder. This now encompasses conditions such as Asperger Syndrome which were not so closely linked under the autism umbrella when Newson was working on PDA. This means that there are individuals who are more "able" who are autistic and have higher demands put on them. Their potentially more subtle presentation of ASD also means these individuals are put in situations where there is higher expectation. They may be attending mainstream schools and don't meet the threshold for EHC plans. This again impacts the pressure to behave as neurotypicals would daily, meaning these children are hardly given a chance to regulate. On the contrary, there are almost constant demands on them with little let-up.

In addition to the stress that parents of children with a PDA presentation are under, there is an increasing number of medical professionals who are offering official private PDA diagnoses. In desperation, numerous parents are paying thousands of pounds to have their children diagnosed in the hope that they will receive the support that they need. The post-PDA diagnosis outcome is often not the one that they had imagined or hoped for. Local authorities that have refused to assess for PDA are not going to suddenly offer support for it once they are given a private assessment. One family Charlotte spoke to paid out for all three of their children to have an official PDA diagnosis. The financial cost was considerable, and the outcome caused them further distress when they were informed by their local authority that none of their children reached the threshold for an EHC plan.

Throughout this family's years of assessment, I was shocked that no NHS clinician or SEND operative had informed the parents that PDA wasn't a recognised or acknowledged diagnosis or that the widely held belief is that PDA is caused by extreme anxiety. This parent became disheartened and frustrated. They were receiving mixed messages and despite their best efforts, they were no further forward. They had lost faith in the system and made a formal complaint against their NHS paediatrician in the hope that they could at least recoup some of the thousands of pounds that they spent on the diagnoses. Their complaint was unsuccessful. The paediatrician had, after all, worked within the currently accepted diagnostic guidance. Unusually, the paediatrician had offered before the children's private assessments to refer the oldest two to their local CAMHs to assess their anxiety. The parent was so focused on PDA that they disregarded this and at the time were unaware of the link between PDA and anxiety.

Not having clear and accessible information for parents puts further and unnecessary pressure on parents and their relationship with professionals. Professionals can sometimes assume that parents should know information that they perceive as "obvious" and see parents search for answers as simply wanting to collect diagnoses.

Even when parents are given advice, the lack of information and support means that there is a difference in opinion. Many parents are told their child needs to be in an environment with no demands. Does such a place even exist? If you managed to find that environment it isn't going to be a lifelong solution. If that child manages to be happy at home, for example, provided they don't have to leave the home, do any chores, schoolwork or any other demands, then they will be fine. What happens when boredom sets in? By this point, the parent has decided that they will remove all demands and doesn't want to reintroduce them. Or, as they discovered in a household with multiple children presenting with PDA, what happens if one child's optimum environment clashes with another child's optimum demand-free environment? There are few obvious or tangible solutions when going down this route.

In PDA the child is avoiding demands by any means they can. Their brain perceives the demand as intolerant. It makes their brains feel dysregulated but, in the same way as a food intolerance versus an allergy, their brains are not allergic to demands. Someone who is gluten intolerant for example may be able to eat a sandwich made with gluten bread and have no major side effects. However, for a person with celiac disease, consuming gluten would have a more severe and detrimental impact. A person with an intolerance learns to manage the intolerance. This may include some exposure to intolerance and strategies to support the impact of the exposure and possibly drug therapy. Telling parents to focus on the removal of demands is treating the symptoms rather than the cause, but they are potentially creating even more anxiety and making the problem worse.

One potentially negative and anxiety-inducing impact of the removal of demands for autistic children is the resulting loss of structure. Structure is a recognised positive for many autistic individuals and has the benefit of dramatically reducing anxiety. By removing demands, the child may no longer demonstrate the avoidant behaviour, but is this helping them in the long term?

Whether we like it or not, demands are an essential component of life. There will always be demands and many of them we could do without. Charlotte is sure she is not alone when she looks at a full basket of laundry demanding to be ironed? Demands take so many forms and some cannot be avoided. For example, if a child needs lifesaving medical interventions, this will most likely contain demands in the form of tests and procedures, some of which may not be pleasant. If a child is not supported in being able to cope with demand then they are being failed.

In the UK when a child turns 16, if they are diagnosed with a learning disability or long-term illness, (which not everyone with ASD or a PDA presentation is) they are likely to undergo a quality of life and dignity assessment. There are 8 areas to the assessment - choice and control, communication, eating, pain management, personal hygiene, practical assistance, privacy and social inclusion. These are believed to be the basic standards required to enable a person to have a good quality of life.

It is a shame that these 8 areas are not considered for all children who are disabled or neurodivergent. If care was focussed around these areas, then so many of the quick-fix ideas suggested by paediatric teams to parents and carers wouldn't be said. In the case of the command of removing demands this could and in Charlotte's experience often impacts upon 7 of the 8 priorities of a quality-of-life assessment. The only one that it meets potentially is choice and control, although if there has been a blanket removal of demands then this may not be within the child's choice or control.

The removal of demands isn't the only generalised solution I have heard about how to help a child with PDA. Another is, "make sure you ask them in the right way". Again this is a very neurotypical solution to a neurodivergent problem. I have seen numerous parents phrase their demands very carefully often with little success. Why? Two reasons.

Firstly, they spend so much time focusing on vocabulary being the key to successful communication, rather than looking at the bigger picture of neurodivergent communication and thinking about the method of communication. This includes the environment that the communication is happening in and most importantly, the current level of regulation for the individual and their ability to process the demand and communicate their response. Whilst this solution is likely to have better outcomes in the long term, the parents/carers and everyone that work with the child must understand in full what is meant by communication.

Secondly, if we examine the widely held belief that PDA is caused by anxiety, then why does it present in the avoidance of demands? In most cases, PDA is seen in individuals who have an autism diagnosis or who are presenting as neurodivergent. A neurotypical person can verbalise their anxiety. For example, if they are anxious about busy shopping centres, they can share this feeling allowing others to understand how they are feeling. For a neurodivergent person, particularly in childhood, expecting them to be able to identify and verbally communicate fear is virtually impossible. In the same way, as we see a meltdown being a response to sensory demands and dysregulation, in PDA the avoidant behaviour isn't behavioural, it is a form of communication they are not coping with.

The presentation of PDA isn't the only way that a neurodivergent individual presents with anxiety. Charlotte doesn't understand her presentation of anxiety. She always works on the assumption that "I am me and I don't attempt to compartmentalise thoughts and behaviours into diagnosis subsections". However, Charlotte has been told that she will often go over and above if someone asks her to do something. She has been told she is a people pleaser, which she finds odd as she doesn't care what most people think of her. There will always be numerous presentations of neurodivergent anxiety.

Charlotte has taught children who have a PDA profile highlighted on their diagnosis. One child was waiting to transfer to a more suitable placement. In the meantime, the SENCO advised staff that the advice from the child's medical team was not to ask the child to do anything. How is that possible in a classroom setting when inclusion should be a paramount consideration in everything you do? It isn't. Even if the teacher decided to follow these instructions, another child would at some point put a demand of some description on the "demand-free" pupil. Charlotte was fortunate that this child liked her subject, music. She was also very aware that their presentation was wide-ranging. Most of her colleagues assumed this was down to the "severity" of their autism. Utter rubbish. It was their anxiety. Their anxiety couldn't be more evident. Even on "good" days, subtle body language cues pointed to anxiety.

Excluding and ignoring a pupil was not going to mitigate their anxiety. If anything, they would feel isolated and potentially more anxious. This was an occasion when communication was key. It wasn't about the way that the demand was presented. It was about delivery and communication. Rather than walking into the class and giving the student a series of demands, Charlotte knew that they liked to have time to process instructions and work in their own order. The class in question were doing a project on film music and had scope for IT and individual work. She made up an envelope for each child. In the envelope, there were a set of cinema tickets. Each one had a different task on it and each task had three levels. By giving each child their own envelopes, their work was differentiated which was a bonus to this method of communication. The child who was "demand free" completed all the tasks to a high standard.

That lunchtime, the teacher who taught that class after Charlotte was discussing their experience. They couldn't believe the child was compliant and did engage with some of the lesson. They said it was as if they were calmer than normal and able to engage.

Charlotte bumped into this child and their parents a few years after they had left their mainstream school. He was in school number two when she met them, and it was a delight to hear that after completing their primary education in a specialist provision they were able to return to mainstream. Their mother told Charlotte that the problem wasn't their autism and ADHD. It was anxiety.

Anxiety is a difficult concept for some people. We are not meaning feeling a little anxious, which let's face it is a part of life and a valid and necessary human emotion. We are referring to anxiety in a clinical term when it moves from being an emotion to being a mental health disorder. We know that in the UK there is a crisis in the care and treatment of mental health, and this could well be one reason why PDA has remained somewhat of an enigma. If there were to be a widespread acknowledgement that demand avoidance was a sign of anxiety and that it was prevalent amongst neurodivergent individuals, children and adolescent mental health services would be overflowing even more than they currently are. There is no infrastructure within the system to cope with this revelation, especially given most CAMHs services will not see individuals with autism unless their mental health difficulties can be proven to be separate from their autism. As PDA, if acknowledged at all, is seen as a trait of autism this would and does mean that currently treatment is even harder to come by.

Charlotte has worked with some children and young people with a PDA profile who have been treated for their anxiety and the difference is incredible. Children who were unable to leave the house or attend school or social occasions are gradually able to. It takes more than anxiolytic medication though and this is another challenge. It takes an understanding of neurodivergent anxiety presentations and most importantly, the way that it presents in that individual. This often comes down to the interventions of the parents and carers. They too can be overwhelmed and the thought of pushing their child out of their comfort zones can be as big an obstacle for the parent as it can be for the child. In many cases, this again comes down to a lack of appropriate support from professionals to explain and encourage parents, and an acknowledgement that it is more than likely the parent will be neurodivergent themselves. They may be anxious to revisit this area as it may bring unwanted and currently extinguished behaviours back.

If we agree that PDA is in essence a presentation of anxiety disorders found in autistic people, then we have a key to getting the correct help. Charlotte's son was first treated by CAMHS when he was 9. Although this was 33 years after the first mention of PDA, it was not a term that was as commonly used as it is now. In hindsight, Pic did demonstrate many of the commonly perceived PDA traits. There were a couple of years when he was not engaging in daily activity and this was in part down to his mental health. It required careful reintegration once his mental health was stabilising and this process was repeated after the Covid pandemic lockdowns.

What is the answer? One which both Danielle and Charlotte's autistic brain constantly craves. Clarity.

Firstly, a clearly defined and accepted definition of PDA. I hope that this would be a trait or presentation of autism. Like being non-verbal or having sensory processing disorder, these are both parts of autism and not standalone diagnoses. A feeling or presentation which is experienced by many autistic people but something that needs highlighting in that person's presentation at a specific time rather than as a separate diagnosis.

One of the arguments frequently used against PDA being linked to autism is that the presentation of PDA entails the use of manipulative behaviours that require a higher level of social understanding than would be found in an autistic person. This is an interesting argument and one which I have considered frequently over the past few years. Is the intention of the individual with PDA to socially manipulate a situation? Or is it simply that their anxiety has reached such a high point that the only response they have left is to refuse to engage with the demand? The chances are the behaviour is being observed by a neurotypical individual who perceives the behaviour to be socially manipulative within society's typical parameters and behaviour structure. Instead, it is as previously mentioned. Demand avoidance is the only way for individuals to communicate their frustration and anxiety.

Secondly, focus on the cause rather than the reaction. Looking at PDA as an atypical presentation of an anxiety disorder and having clear treatment and support routes. Giving parents and carers clear advice about how best to support their child. Not just blanket phrases which are open to misinterpretation. Ensuring that everyone who works with that child is using the same techniques so as not to cause further anxiety by having a different approach.

Thirdly, not dismissing the use of carefully monitored anxiolytic medication to reduce and stabilise the individual's anxiety so that they can process demands. Alongside medication would be a specialised form of CBT which would be individualised to consider the person's level of communication, anxiety and cognitive functioning. If communication is a major consideration, then this needs to be done in conjunction with speech and language therapists.

Fourthly, supporting parents to understand ways to help their child to overcome some of their anxiety. Explaining the importance of ensuring that they can mitigate as many of the PDA traits as possible to ensure that they live a happy and positive life. Also, explain that whilst autism is a lifelong diagnosis and is different. A person can experience different autistic traits and symptoms at different intensities at different times.

It is important to never underestimate the importance of parental support and education. This does need to be gauged appropriately and to make sure that they are not feeling as if they are being given parenting classes. Having a child with PDA will most likely result in them having experienced many embarrassing situations, leaving them feeling quite vulnerable. Whilst the parents' feelings need to be taken into account, it is important for the child's welfare and outcomes that they are told if there are things they are doing which might be harming their child.

Whilst clarity is important, it is also important to acknowledge that autism is not a behavioural disorder and there is nothing to stop an autistic person from having a separate diagnosis of a behavioural disorder. If exploring the anxiety route doesn't have the desired impact, then the possibility of a behavioural disorder mustn't be dismissed without due consideration.

The PDA question will one day be resolved. How and when remains unclear. What is important is that it does not become a trend, an excuse for lazy parenting or an obstacle that isn't acknowledged by professionals meaning that the outcomes for the child are impacted. Most importantly, whilst there is no clear guidance for assessment and diagnosis, private healthcare professionals should not take advantage of the vulnerable position that parents find themselves in and take money for diagnosing the undiagnosable.

CHAPTER TEN

Tips on supporting your child

There are no quick fixes for anxiety. As we explained in the first chapter, some of us, regardless of any neuro divergence, are more prone to anxiety due to our brain's genetic makeup. This means that whilst there might be triggers for anxiety the chances are that person would be pre-dispositioned to anxiety regardless of the situation.

While you as the parent and carer arm yourself with as much knowledge about anxiety as possible, with various solutions that might help, it's important you don't look for comparisons between your child's anxiety and anyone else's presentation. This includes your own if you have clinical anxiety.

A positive approach

Anxiety impacts the entire family and having a child or family member with a clinical anxiety disorder is not easy. However, the one thing that won't help your child to overcome their anxiety is letting yourself feel negative too. Being positive and encouraging means that your child's self-esteem is also boosted and that too can have a positive impact on their recovery.

By all means take time for yourself to feel and express the stress you are feeling, whether through counselling or friends and family. However, do not do this in front of your child. It will not help them understand more and only lowers their self-worth and determination to overcome the anxiety they are feeling.

The road to recovery

In the same way that everyone is impacted by anxiety individually, their road to recovery will also be unique. Ownership of this journey is important, and it can help them to realise that recovery does not happen in a straight line. They will most likely feel as though they are on a roundabout, with the feeling that they keep returning to their original starting point and not making the progress you or they had hoped or thought.

In time you can exit that roundabout, and the journey may still not be on a straight road but there will be fewer twists and turns. It's very possible that a relapse can occur, and at these times it is important to reassure them that they have made progress before. It is just a temporary setback.

Communication takes all forms

Traditional talking therapies are very hit-and-miss when it comes to autistic people, though there are an increasing amount of CBT options which are adapted for neurodivergent people. These can be hard to access and are still not right for everyone.

What is essential to understand anxiety, is that you learn to express it. Self-expression can come in many forms including:

- Poetry
- Writing Prose
- Art
- Music
- Playing
- Baking
- Sport and Fitness

Expression is about having an outlet where you can express your fears and find solutions. You may be able to find out what an anxiety trigger is by watching your child play or draw. They might act out their anxieties to help process them. Using alternative methods of expression and communication can help you find the cause and also work through solutions and reassure.

When Charlotte was 14, she wrote about how music made her feel and helped her process her anxiety.

"Words are arduous and a gruelling way to communicate. I can't put it into words how my head feels inside. Emotions good and bad are best processed through music. The transpicuous clarity with which my brain can process even the darkest thoughts gives me an instant respite from the turmoils of my inner self. My worries may inhabit my head but quickly evacuate my body as my fingers touch the keys of the piano. At times it is as if Mozart shared the polar experiences of my brain. His solemn adagios allow an out pouring before my brain resets with his Rondo Alla Turca or his Sonata in D."

For Charlotte, spoken words were difficult to use in expressing her emotions. Through her music however, she was able to feel and express how she felt.

Quite often, the person suffering from anxiety won't realise they are expressing their fears or feelings. When Danielle was 18, she studied for her Art A-level course. The original theme was 'body art'. You could take it anywhere you wanted to go. It wasn't until several years later, Danielle looked back through her work and realised that she had somehow travelled from an unrelated title to exploring the experience of emotional pain. Her final pieces were an accurate reflection of how she felt at the time when her anxiety was at its worst. When showing her mum, her mum explained that she saw what was happening as she was painting and drawing and that Danielle just needed to be left to express the feelings she didn't even really know she had. It was cathartic and allowed emotions to be freed without any explosive repercussions.

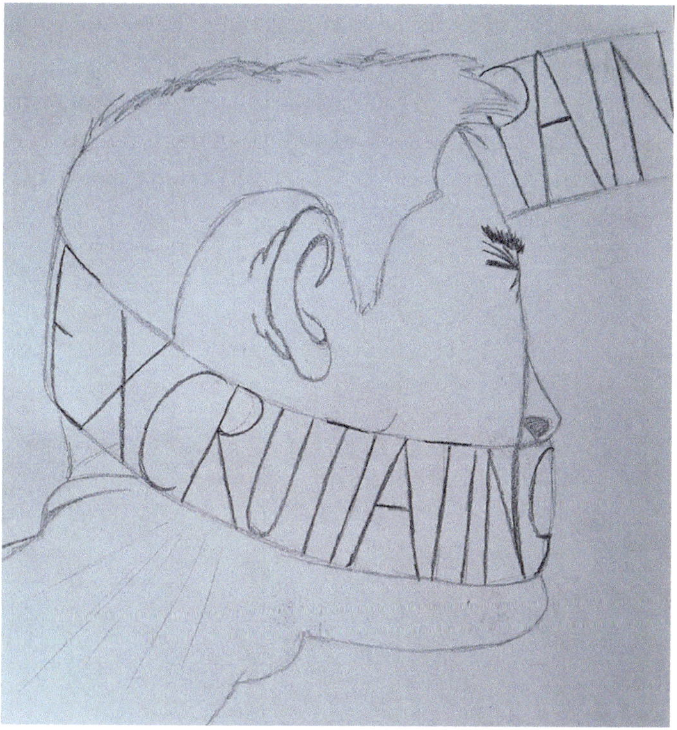

Drawing by Danielle when she was 18, unaware that her feelings were reflected in her artwork.

Act quickly

The autistic brain is rigid, somebody once said to me their autistic child "liked what they know and knows what they like". If an experience is negative that is only going to make their brain even more rigid and they will end up refusing things. In the autistic mind refusing one thing means that things can spiral into so many other areas of their lives as there is a chain reaction. It is important that anxiety is dealt with quickly.

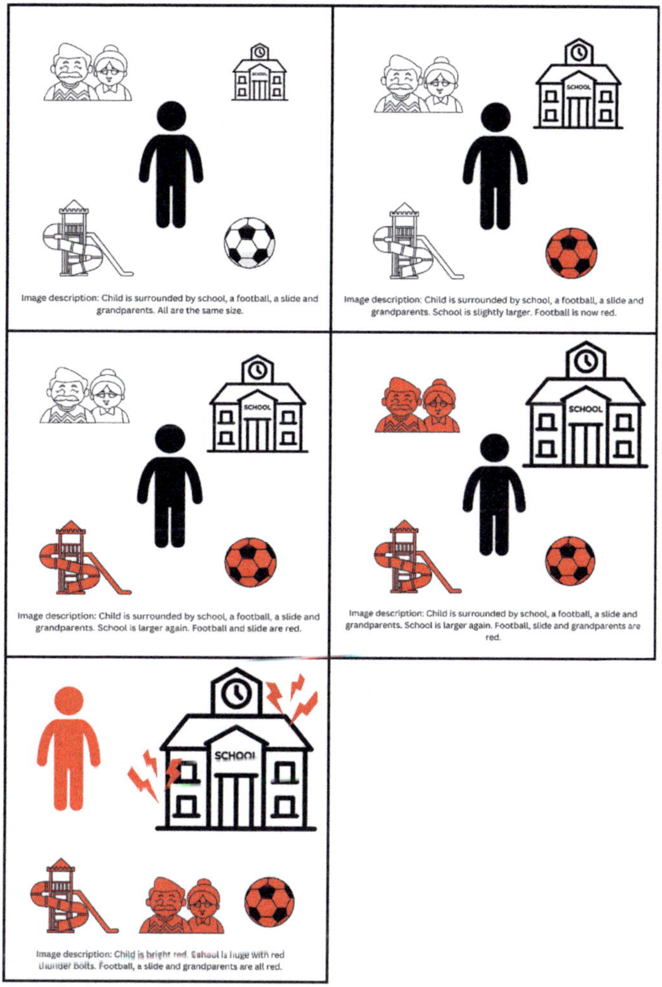
SCHOOL
Image description: Child is surrounded by school, a football, a slide and grandparents. All are the same size.
SCHOOL
Image description: Child is surrounded by school, a football, a slide and grandparents. School is slightly larger. Football is now red.
SCHOOL
Image description: Child is surrounded by school, a football, a slide and grandparents. School is larger again. Football and slide are red.
SCHOOL
Image description: Child is surrounded by school, a football, a slide and grandparents. School is larger again. Football, slide and grandparents are red.
SCHOOL
Image description: Child is bright red. School is huge with red thunder bolts. Football, a slide and grandparents are all red.

As this picture shows, the anxiety about school has spread as the child is unable to resolve their anxiety around school and it quickly begins to affect other areas of life.

Ask for help

Make sure that any professionals working with your child are aware of their anxiety. It is important to give factual accounts of how their anxiety presents and what you think the triggers are. Don't be tempted to use words such as "crippling" or "severe" as such descriptions tend to be lost as they are not clinical descriptions or your child's descriptions, but your perception.

It is also important to keep a clear diary of what you see so that can be given to the professional at the meeting.

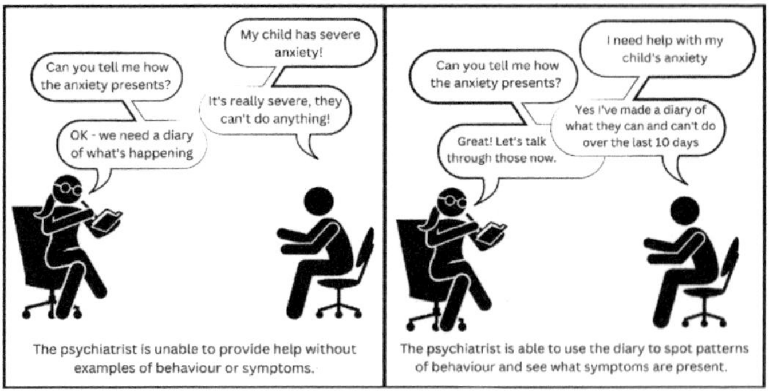
My child has severe anxiety!
Can you tell me how the anxiety presents?
It's really severe, they can't do anything!
OK - we need a diary of what's happening
I need help with my child's anxiety
Can you tell me how the anxiety presents?
Yes I've made a diary of what they can and can't do over the last 10 days
Great! Let's talk through those now.

The psychiatrist is unable to provide help without examples of behaviour or symptoms.

The psychiatrist is able to use the diary to spot patterns of behaviour and see what symptoms are present.

Medication

Some people with anxiety need medication. This isn't an instant fix. In the UK anti-anxiety medication can only be prescribed by a child and adolescent psychiatrist and they will need a referral to this service. Each trust has its criteria for treatment and acceptance of the service as well as referral routes. Medication needs to be discussed carefully with the professional to make sure that it is the correct route for your child. If your child is old enough and able, they will be included in the discussions too.

Make it worth their while to change a thought process

One of the lasting effects of anxiety which is experienced by neurodivergent children is a learnt response. This can occur even after they have started to work through their anxiety or have had a therapeutic or medical intervention. Once your child is ready to start to "face their fears" and overcome this automatic learnt response, you need to make it worth their while.

This doesn't mean you are going to be buying lots of expensive treats. It doesn't even have to be a purchased treat. It could be a shared activity, extra screen time, a new book or if appropriate a purchased item. We are not saying that you shouldn't buy something, but we want to show that it is possible to get a similar effect without spending a fortune, or anything at all.

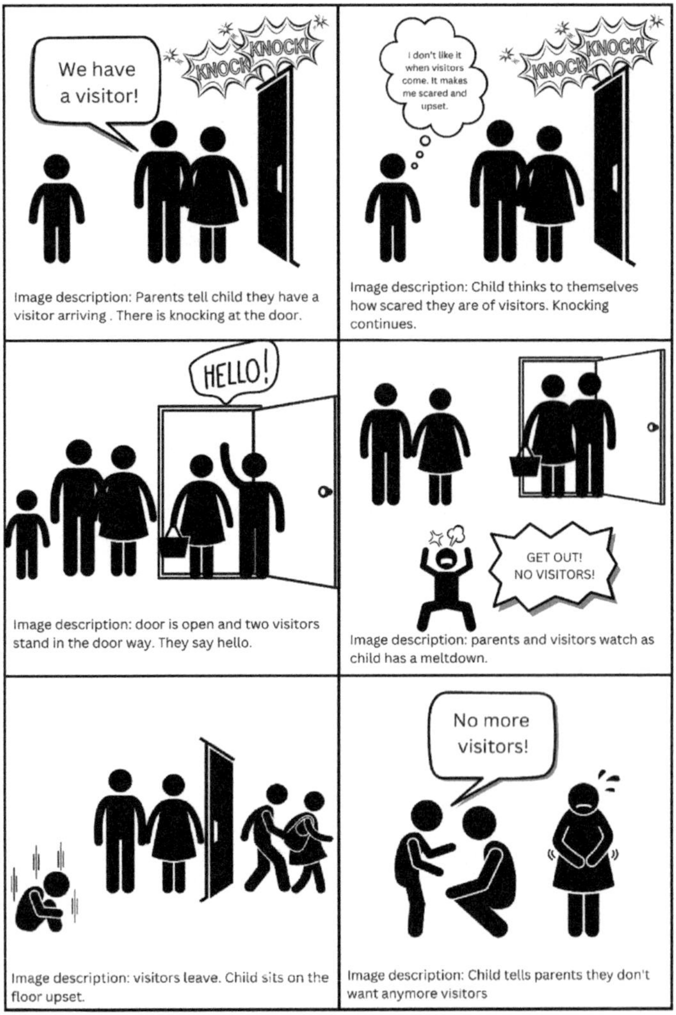

Image description: Parents tell child they have a visitor arriving . There is knocking at the door.

Image description: Child thinks to themselves how scared they are of visitors. Knocking continues.

Image description: door is open and two visitors stand in the door way. They say hello.

Image description: parents and visitors watch as child has a meltdown.

Image description: visitors leave. Child sits on the floor upset.

Image description: Child tells parents they don't want anymore visitors

Although the child had overcome a lot of their anxieties, their brain followed the routine that they had become used to. By adding an incentive, it changes the brain pattern.

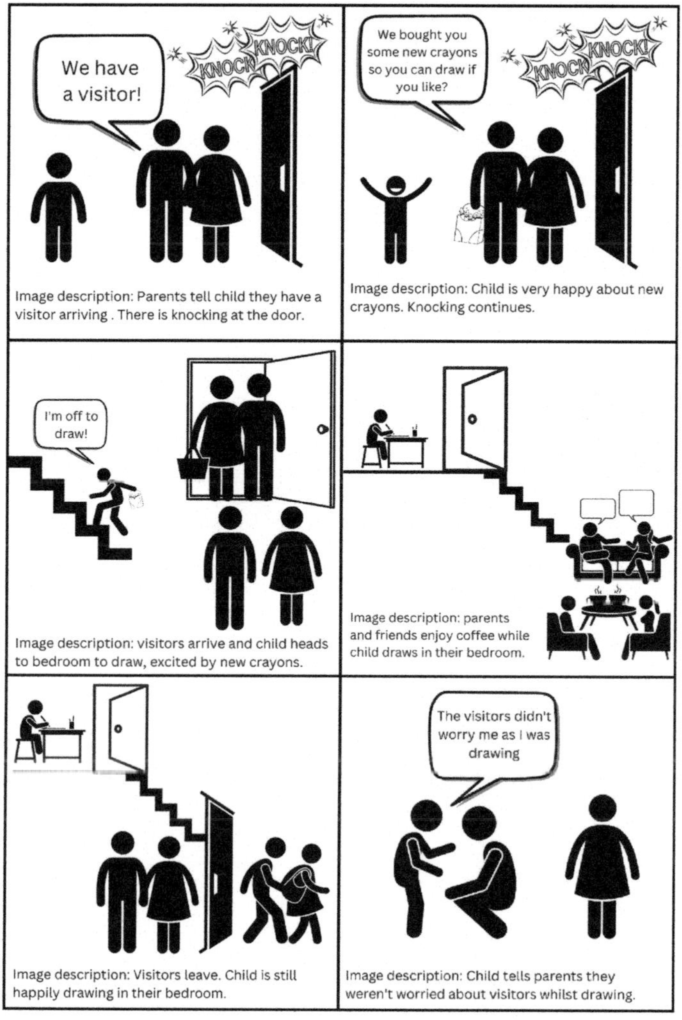

The small change, the child hasn't had much interaction with their visitor but the experience is positive. This means they can gradually change their brain's picture of what having a visitor is like.

Don't use confusing phrases

A lot of neurodivergent children are literal thinkers. Using social stories can help but be careful to avoid terms such as "butterflies in your tummy". When this was said to me as a child I was terrified. I was no longer concerned about the activity I was anxious about but by the thought I had loads of real butterflies inside me.

Some children will be able to understand this but make sure your effort to help them doesn't backfire.

Finally, what your child needs is patience, understanding and compassion. Respect what they find anxiety provoking and work through it with them. Just because it doesn't make sense to you, doesn't mean it isn't hugely significant for them.